LECTURE NOTES ON GASTROENTEROLOGY

LECTURE NOTES ON
GASTROENTEROLOGY

RICHARD D. TONKIN
M.D., F.R.C.P.
Consultant Physician
Westminster Hospital, London

AND

J. A. PARRISH
M.D., M.R.C.P.
Consultant Physician
Mayday Hospital, Croydon
Honorary Clinical Assistant
St. Mark's Hospital, London

BLACKWELL SCIENTIFIC PUBLICATIONS
OXFORD AND EDINBURGH

© BLACKWELL SCIENTIFIC PUBLICATIONS 1968

This book is copyright. It may not be reproduced in whole or in part without permission. Application with regard to copyright should be addressed to the publisher.

SBN 632 04090 4

FIRST PUBLISHED IN 1968

Printed in Great Britain by
WATMOUGHS LIMITED, IDLE, BRADFORD; AND LONDON
and bound by
THE KEMP HALL BINDERY, OXFORD

CONTENTS

	Preface	vii
1	The Oesophagus	1
2	The Stomach	14
3	Indigestion	22
4	Peptic Ulcer	26
5	Acute Gastro-intestinal Bleeding	34
6	The Liver	39
7	The Biliary Tract	64
8	The Pancreas	72
9	The Small Intestine	83
10	The Malabsorption Syndrome	96
11	Anaemia and the Alimentary Tract	101
12	Intestinal Infections	106
13	Helminth Infestations	120
14	Diarrhoea	130
15	Regional Entero-colitis	143

Contents

16	The Colon and Rectum	148
17	Ulcerative Colitis	158
18	Rarer Gastro-intestinal Conditions	167
19	Investigation Techniques	178
20	Diet	192
	Examination Questions	197
	Recommended Books of Reference	202
	Index	203

PREFACE

Gastroenterology is a rapidly expanding subject and in recent years the literature in the field has become extensive.

This book has been written with the aim of providing the undergraduate student with a simple classified framework of gastrointestinal disorders on which he or she can build from clinical experience.

In a book of this size it is not possible to describe in detail all the available investigations nor to adjudicate between the inevitable differences of opinion on treatment. It has been necessary to be didactic in order to be concise but the views expressed are those most generally accepted not only in this country but throughout the world.

It is helpful for the student to practise written examinations and in consequence a selection of questions which have been set in recent years is included at the end of the book. We would like to take the opportunity to thank the several authorities concerned for permission to reproduce questions from their examination papers.

R.D.T.
J.A.P.

CHAPTER 1

THE OESOPHAGUS

The following disorders are discussed in this chapter:
  Oesophagitis
  Hiatus hernia
  Achalasia
  Carcinoma
  Oesophageal varices
  Congenital anomalies
  Diverticula
  Trauma
  Foreign bodies

OESOPHAGITIS

Classification
  1 **Acute (corrosive)**
  2 **Subacute**
  3 **Chronic (atrophic)**
  4 **Recurrent (reflux)**

1 Acute Corrosive Oesophagitis

Aetiology

This emergency arises from the accidental or suicidal swallowing of corrosive fluids.

Clinical features

The patient will have burns and inflammation of the lips, tongue and mouth, severe retrosternal pain and may be in a state of shock.

Treatment

In the early stages immediate inactivation of the corrosive agent, antibiotics and intravenous feeding are needed. If the patient survives, strictures may develop as a result of scarring. Steroids may be given in the healing phase to try and lessen fibrous tissue formation.

2 Subacute Oesophagitis

Aetiology

The pharynx and oesophagus become inflamed due to mucosal infections arising:
- (a) because of a lack of effective polymorphonuclear leucocytes in
  - (i) toxic granulopaenia i.e. glandular fever
  - (ii) leukaemia
- (b) because of an alteration in bacterial flora in long term broad spectrum antibiotic therapy.

Clinical features

The patient complains of dysphagia and will have an inflamed pharynx. There will be a white exudate in cases of monilial infection.

Investigations

1. A pharyngeal swab culture may demonstrate the responsible organism.
2. A differential white count may reveal granulopaenia or leukaemia.
3. A Barium swallow X-ray may show a characteristic irregular oesophageal outline.

Treatment

In the first group oral hygiene, together with an antibiotic will help.

In the second group withdrawal of the broad spectrum antibiotic and substitution with Nystatin or Amphotericin is necessary.

3 Chronic Atrophic Oesophagitis

Aetiology

The atrophy is due to chronic iron deficiency and the term Sideropaenic Dysphagia is preferable to either of the eponyms Patterson Kelly or Plummer Vinson syndrome since it defines the aetiology and symptoms.

Pathology

The mucosa in this condition is thin and smooth and the submucosa infiltrated with inflammatory cells. Sometimes a thin vascularised membrane develops from the anterior wall of the oesophagus, the so-called 'web'.

Clinical features

The presenting symptom is dysphagia and care must be taken not to confuse the diagnosis with either 'globus hystericus', a psychological condition, or with carcinoma.

Treatment

Prolonged treatment with oral iron in high dosage (600 mg. three times a day) is usually effective but parenteral iron may occasionally be necessary.

4 Recurrent Reflux Oesophagitis

Aetiology

As its name implies, the inflammatory reaction results from the action of the regurgitated gastric juice on the mucosa of the lower third of the oesophagus which, unlike the gastric mucosa, has no natural defence against acid. It is important to recognise that an hiatus hernia need *not* be present, the regurgitation in these patients being a physiological dysfunction.

Other causative factors:

1. Gastric hypersecretion.
2. Associated lesions such as a duodenal ulcer or cholecystitis.
3. Chronic anxiety and nervous strain.
4. Mechanical factors causing a raised intra-abdominal pressure such as obesity, tight clothing or bending.

Pathology

Persistent acid regurgitation will always give rise to distal oesophagitis and although this is reversible in the early stages may progress to ulceration and fibrous stricture formation if allowed to continue.

A *peptic* ulcer of the oesophagus (Barrett's ulcer) can only occur when the lower few centimetres of the oesophagus are lined by gastric mucosa as may be seen in a sliding hiatus hernia or as a congenital anomaly.

Clinical features

Deep substernal discomfort, usually described as heartburn, is the characteristic symptom. This is aggravated by stooping or bending and by lying down at night.

Not infrequently there is actual regurgitation of stomach contents.

Investigations

1. Oesophagoscopy will show the inflammation of the lower oesophagus.
2. Barium meal and screening will demonstrate reflux into the oesophagus.

Treatment

The following measures are aimed at diminishing the gastro-oesophageal reflux and reducing the acidity of the gastric contents:

1. Small frequent, regular meals.
2. Consistent antacid medication.
3. Elevation of the head of the bed at night.
4. Weight reduction where needed.
5. Avoiding bending or tight corsets.

Such treatment will permit resolution of the oesophagitis in the majority of cases.

HIATUS HERNIA

Classification

1 Sliding hernia
2 Rolling hernia

The Oesophagus

Pathology

1. The sliding type is commoner and consists of a cuff of stomach protruding through the hiatus into the chest, the cardio-oesophageal junction thus coming to lie above the level of the diaphragm.
2. In the rolling type there is a pouch of stomach protruding up alongside the oesophagus into the chest, the cardio-oesophageal junction remaining in its normal position.

Hiatus hernia should not be confused with eventration of the diaphragm, a congenital anomaly in which the diaphragm consists of a functionless fibrous membrane. True eventration is usually left-sided and rarely gives rise to symptoms.

Clinical features

1. The sliding hernia is usually, but not invariably, associated with reflux and oesophagitis.
2. The rolling hernia is less consistently associated with reflux but may give rise to localised low substernal discomfort.
3. Both types are usually spontaneously reducible in the erect position and it is important to recognise that neither need be the cause of any symptoms. On the other hand if the hernia becomes fixed, then symptoms are more likely to be persistent.
4. Either may be associated with anaemia due to recurrent blood loss.

Investigations

1. Plain X-ray of the chest may suggest a large hernia.
2. Barium swallow and meal will confirm the presence of the hernia.

Treatment

The principles of medical management are identical with those described for uncomplicated reflux oesophagitis and these measures, particularly weight control, should be given a thorough trial before advising surgical correction.

Surgery is indicated where:
  (a) There are complications such as
    (i) stricture formation in a sliding hernia

6 *Lecture Notes on Gastroenterology*

(ii) cardiac or pulmonary distress due to the size of a rolling hernia

(b) Symptoms make life intolerable and medical treatment has failed to control them.

ACHALASIA OF THE CARDIA

Aetiology

In this condition there is a disturbance of oesophagael motility, the most important feature being a failure of the distal ampullary segment of the oesophagus to relax on the arrival of a bolus of food.

The basic defect in achalasia is probably either a diminution of the total number of ganglion cells of the intramural autonomic nerve plexuses or an impairment of their normal pharmacological activity.

Pathology

The body of the oesophagus becomes dilated, partly as a result of the defect in its activity and partly because of the constant retention of food. The cardio-oesophageal junction remains closed and although there is no actual spasm, persistence of the background muscle tone effectively prevents entry of the residual column of food into the stomach except in very small amounts.

An acquired form of the condition is found in Chaga's disease or endemic mega-oesophagus occurring in Brazil, in which infestation by Trypanosoma cruzi causes destruction of the ganglion cells.

Clinical features

The characteristic symptom is post-prandial lower substernal discomfort with subsequent regurgitation of unchanged food. The regurgitated fluid is always alkaline in reaction, which distinguishes it from gastric regurgitation.

The condition predisposes to inter-current pulmonary infection due to spill-over of the oesophageal food reservoir.

Investigations

1 A straight chest film may provide the diagnosis since the

The Oesophagus

symptomatic control of inoperative cases. Where resection is not possible, intubation down the oesophagus through the tumour area may be employed as a temporary palliative measure and is almost always preferable to establishing a gastrostomy.

OESOPHAGEAL VARICES

Aetiology

The cardio-oesophageal junction is a major site of communications between the portal and systemic venous systems and varicose distension at this point is the inevitable sequel to a sustained rise in the portal venous pressure.

Pathology

The causes of portal hypertension are obstruction of the portal vein or its branches

   (i) in the liver
   (ii) in the portal hepatis
   (iii) in its abdominal course.

All types of intra-hepatic fibrosis result in time in increased portal pressure although the commonest is multilobular (Laennec's) cirrhosis.

Enlargement of lymph nodes, particularly due to malignancy, in the portal fissure causes obstruction of either the portal vein or the bile duct but in spite of the common occurrence of such glands, obstruction is relatively infrequent.

The portal vein in its course across the posterior abdominal wall may become obstructed by external pressure or may become thrombosed. Frequently the cause of the thrombosis is not obvious.

Clinical features

Oesophageal varices are symptomless until they bleed but when they do, the presenting symptom is usually an effortless haematemesis. Occasionally no blood is vomited, in which case melaena may be the only evidence of bleeding.

Investigations

1 A Barium swallow should be carried out to confirm the diagnosis.
2 Oesophagoscopy is helpful if there is doubt.

When bleeding comes from varices in the fundus of the stomach, then differentiation from a bleeding peptic ulcer may be surprisingly difficult.

Treatment

The immediate needs are:
  (a) Management of the associated shock
  (b) Control of haemorrhage
  (c) Blood replacement.

Posterior pituitary extract (20 units in 200 ml of saline i.v.) may reduce bleeding by constricting the splanchnic arterioles thereby lowering portal venous pressure.

When bleeding persists the insertion of an oesophago-gastric balloon may be necessary (Sengstaken tube). This achieves control by internal pressure on the distended veins in the fundus of the stomach as well as those in the lower oesophagus. Having controlled the haemorrhage it becomes equally important to clear the gut of blood by means of gastric lavage and aperients in order to lessen the risk of hepatic coma.

Subsequently in order to forestall a recurrence, the advisability of surgery has to be considered. Diversion of the portal venous flow by means of a porta-caval or lieno-renal anastomosis or elimination of the collateral veins by gastric transection are the procedures employed.

Transection of the upper part of the stomach and ligation of the veins can be undertaken as an emergency procedure.

CONGENITAL ANOMALIES

Pathology

The anomalies are various degrees of atresia from simple stricture to absence of segments or of fistulous communications with the respiratory passages.

The Oesophagus

Clinical features

Most of these disorders present within a few hours or days of birth because of excessive pharyngeal mucus and feeding and respiratory difficulties.

Treatment

Surgical correction is needed but early diagnosis is essential so that temporary feeding methods can be introduced and the infant can get established before definitive surgery is undertaken.

DIVERTICULA

Aetiology

These may develop as a result of external fibrosis and scarring (traction diverticula) or from internal pressure on a weak, possibly congenital, point in the oesophageal muscle wall (pulsion diverticula).

Clinical features

Most oesophageal diverticula are entirely symptom free but occasionally an intermittent type of dysphagia may be experienced.

Treatment

Intractable symptoms demand surgical resection which can prove a hazardous procedure.

TRAUMA

Aetiology

Because of its anatomical situation the oesophagus is well protected against external injury but damage can occur after:
1 A severe epigastric impact, such as may be delivered by the steering wheel of a car resulting in rupture of the lower segment with or without the production of a traumatic diaphragmatic hernia.

2 Attempts to suppress vomiting.
3 Forceful retching, for example following alcoholic excess, causing a linear rupture of the mucous membrane and haematemesis (the Mallory-Weiss syndrome).
4 Instrumentation. This is more likely in the elderly patient and especially when cervical osteo-phytosis is present. It may result from prolonged pressure by the instrument as well as from direct instrument tip trauma.

Clinical features

There may be:

1 Surgical emphysema in the neck.
2 Signs of mediastinitis with retrosternal discomfort and fever.
3 Signs of fluid and irritation of the pleura.
4 Dysphagia.

but it is important to remember that such injuries need not result in obvious immediate signs and symptoms as these may occur up to forty-eight hours later.

Investigations

If there is doubt about the diagnosis, a small quantity of lipiodol taken by mouth may demonstrate the oesophageal tear.

Treatment

1 Allow no food or fluid by mouth.
2 Pass a high oesophageal tube to aspirate mouth and pharyngeal secretions.
3 Give antibiotics.
4 Carry out surgical repair wherever possible.

FOREIGN BODIES

Aetiology

Foreign bodies present a problem in children who swallow parts of toys and other objects they try to taste. In adults fish or small animal bones are more usually to blame. The majority of such objects pass rapidly into the stomach but when impaction occurs in the oesophagus, the situation is potentially dangerous and should be treated as an emergency.

Clinical features

The patient usually presents with deep substernal discomfort and dysphagia but it is important to recognise that he need not have any knowledge of the entrance of the foreign body.

Treatment

Immediate radiological investigation of all suspected cases is essential, followed by oesophagoscopy for confirmation and if possible removal. Every hour the foreign body remains *in situ* decreases the chance of locating it in the surrounding inflammatory reaction and increases the risk of serious complications such as perforation, mediastinitis and empyema.

CHAPTER 2

THE STOMACH

The commoner abnormalities in the stomach are:
>   **Gastritis**
>   **Peptic Ulcer (see Chapter 4)**
>   **Malignant Tumours**
>   **Hypertrophic Pyloric Stenosis**
>   **Diverticula**
>   **Volvulus**

GASTRITIS

Classification

1. Acute erosive
2. Sub-acute inflammatory
3. Chronic hypertrophic
4. Chronic atrophic

1 Acute Erosive Gastritis

Pathology

A general inflammatory reaction of the gastric mucosa will occur in response to a sufficiently vigorous stimulus but it is usually transient.

Occasionally a localised area is more severely affected resulting in mucosal erosion with the risk of haemorrhage.

Aetiology

Common examples occur after:
1. A 'celebration', alcohol being a powerful gastric secretory stimulus as well as a direct mucosal irritant.

The Stomach

2 Taking aspirin. While insoluble aspirin is more likely to produce localised inflammation, the more soluble varieties are by no means without risk.
3 Many other drugs in common use are well recognised as gastric irritants, including colchicine, butazolidin, digitalis, aminophylline, emetine and the glucogenic steroids.

Clinical features

Apart from the potential risk of haemorrhages, acute gastritis is not a serious clinical problem and at the most causes mild epigastric discomfort.

Treatment

Simple measures such as withdrawal of the irritant, a bland diet and a short course of antacids are all that are required but if there is a specific drug that cannot be withdrawn or reduced, then it should be given with food or in milk together with an antacid or, if available, in enteric coated form (e.g. prednisolone salazopyrine, etc.)

2 Sub-acute Inflammatory Gastritis

Aetiology

It is important to recognise that a more persistent type of gastritis can occur and is more likely to be encountered in people who habitually enjoy seasoned foods.

Clinical features

The symptoms are similar to those produced by a peptic ulcer, the discomfort taking the form of an epigastric burning sensation.

Differential diagnosis

It may be difficult to distinguish this condition from peptic ulcer and many of the so-called 'X-ray negative' dyspepsias are almost certainly instances of this simple mucosal inflammatory reaction involving the stomach and/or duodenum i.e. 'gastro-duodenitis'.

Investigations

Gastroscopy may demonstrate patchy inflamed areas in the mucosa.

Treatment

As for peptic ulceration with small, frequent regular meals, antacids and antispasmodics.

3 Chronic Hypertrophic Gastritis

Classification
- (a) Hypertrophy of glandular element
- (b) Hypertrophy of epithelial element

- (a) Glandular Hypertrophy.

  This is the most common type and is accompanied by an increase in acid output. There may be mucosal ulceration and occasionally frank bleeding.

  Some patients may be symptomless, others will have abdominal discomfort or pain.

- (b) Epithelial Hypertrophy.

  This has similar macroscopic appearances and some cases have a high protein loss from the mucosa resulting in hypoproteinaemia and oedema (Menetrier's disease).

Investigations
1. Gastroscopy
2. Barium meal X-rays

These will show hypertrophy of the gastric mucosal folds if there is a sufficient increase in the parietal cell mass.

Treatment

In the first group treatment as for peptic ulceration is usually effective. However in rare instances of either types of hypertrophy an extensive or total gastrectomy may be required to reduce either the acid output or the protein loss.

4 Chronic Atrophic Gastritis

Aetiology

Atrophy may occur:
1. In pernicious anaemia when there is atrophy of the mucosa of the body with achylia and loss of intrinsic factor.

The Stomach

2 In old age where some degree of gastric mucosal atrophy is almost invariable.
3 In iron deficiency anaemia particularly in elderly patients suffering from a general malnutrition.
4 After irradiation to the stomach. Deep X-ray therapy was at one time used in cases of peptic ulcer to reduce the secretory capacity.

Pathology

In these patients the stomach has a smooth attenuated mucous membrane with a reduced capacity to produce an acid juice.

Clinical features

Although this condition is not uncommon it rarely gives rise to any symptoms.

Treatment

1 This consists of ensuring a nutritious diet with supplementary oral or parenteral iron.
2 Parenteral vitamin B_{12} and folic acid are also indicated where specific deficiencies have been demonstrated.

MALIGNANT TUMOURS

Carcinoma

Aetiology

1 The sex incidence shows a 2:1 preponderance of males contrasting with the higher incidence of gastric ulcer in women.
2 The maximum age incidence is in the later decades but gastric cancer is by no means unknown in the young.
3 Patients with pernicious anaemia or atrophic gastritis, and also those who have had a partial gastrectomy are more likely to develop carcinoma.

Pathology

The antrum, lesser curve and gastro-oesophageal junction are the commonest sites but no part of the stomach is exempt.

The majority of carcinomas are of the adenomatous mucus-secreting type. These are usually proliferative and have a fungating appearance. Sometimes however they are predominantly infiltrative and appear as large ulcers with rolled edges. Linitis plastica is an extreme form of this infiltrative type in which there may be no obvious breach of the surface mucosa and in which microscopy shows a scirrhous pattern.

Metastasis is by direct extension to neighbouring structures and by lymphatic channels to the regional nodes, including that above the inner end of the left clavicle (Virchow's node). Dissemination by the blood stream is initially to the liver but becomes widespread into lungs, bones, brain and even the skin.

Clinical features

1 Anorexia is the most consistent symptom but is also common in many other conditions. Nevertheless when it is the sole symptom in the older age group the possibility of gastric neoplasm should always be suspected.

Other symptoms are:
2 Weight loss.
3 General malaise.
4 Abdominal discomfort and pain.
5 Symptoms of anaemia, but unfortunately these all too often indicate metastatic spread.

Investigations

1 Barium meal X-rays will reveal the majority of lesions, tumours showing as filling defects or as ulcers. Infiltrating lesions may be detected on screening by observing decreased mobility of the gastric wall.
2 Gastroscopy will show the majority of tumours in the pyloric antrum and body of the stomach but those in the cardia are extremely difficult to see. A biopsy taken under direct vision may confirm the diagnosis but in cases where there is surrounding oedema and inflammation, differen-

tiation between peptic ulcer and cancer may still prove difficult.
3 Exfoliative cytology. In experienced hands examination of cells obtained by gasric washings can be helpful but infiltrating tumours do not always exfoliate into the stomach and false negative results may be obtained.
4 Gastric function tests. These are of limited value for although a low acid output is usual, a normal or even high level does not exclude cancer. Conversely, hypochlorhydria is of frequent occurrence in the absence of any malignant change.

Treatment

There is as yet no effective medical therapy for gastric cancer and early surgery offers the only hope for these patients. Earlier diagnosis is essential if the present unsatisfactory five year survival rate of approximately 10% is to be bettered.

Sarcoma (rare)

The majority of these are lymphosarcomas and the gastric lesion is usually part of a widespread condition.

Occasionally, solitary lymphomas may be encountered and total gastrectomy carries a fair prognosis. The condition is usually radio-sensitive so that post-operative irradiation may help prevent recurrence.

Chemotherapy with one of the nitrogen mustards can be used as an alternative post-operatively.

HYPERTROPHIC PYLORIC STENOSIS

Aetiology

1 Although essentially a condition of infants or children, this congenital anomaly may occasionally present in adult life. There is however not the same male predominance as in the infantile type.
2 Some cases may be secondary to a persistent duodenal or pyloric canal ulcer.

Clinical features

Persistent vomiting is the main symptom and on examination a succussion splash can usually be elicited.

Investigations

Barium meal demonstrates narrowing of the pylorus with some degree of obstruction and the appearances are liable to be misinterpreted as carcinoma.

Treatment

Being benign it requires no more than a pyloroplasty for the relief of symptoms. A full thickness section should always be taken for histology and some surgeons prefer to carry out a pylorectomy to be certain of not missing a carcinoma.

GASTRIC DIVERTICULA

These may be congenital or acquired:
1. Congenital diverticula are of little clinical importance and rarely give rise to symptoms.
2. The majority of acquired diverticula are due to gastric deformity occurring as a result of fibrosis following peptic ulceration.

VOLVULUS OF THE STOMACH

Aetiology

This is an unusual event and may or may not be associated with other gastric disease.

Clinical features

1. The stomach rotates on its long axis and gives rise to sudden attacks of severe epigastric pain radiating through to the back.

The Stomach

2 Retching is more in evidence than vomiting as the cardio-oesophageal junction is usually occluded and swallowed food or fluid is almost immediately rejected.
3 Epigastric distension may be dramatic.

Treatment

Most cases resolve spontaneously without any specific treatment but surgical correction of the condition may be necessary if the attacks are either unduly frequent or very severe.

CHAPTER 3

INDIGESTION

The term indigestion or dyspepsia should properly be reserved for symptoms that are in some way related to the taking of food and of these pain, flatulence, heartburn, acid regurgitation and nausea or vomiting are the commonest.

Indigestion however does not always indicate dysfunction or disease of the gastro-intestinal tract and symptoms of such widely varying conditions as pregnancy, cerebral tumour, renal failure or coronary insufficiency are frequently described by the patient as indigestion and may lead to misinterpretation. In making a diagnosis therefore it is of the utmost importance that the patient not only gives a detailed description of his dyspepsia but also of other symptoms however irrelevant they may at first appear. Similarly examination of the abdomen is often unhelpful but full general examination frequently reveals other underlying conditions.

The following purely clinical classification is useful in differential diagnosis:

Varieties of indigestion:

    1 Painful
    2 Flatulent
    3 Regurgitant
    4 Nauseous
    5 Anorexic
    6 Exertional

1 Painful Indigestion

In this type the pain is generally related to a definite focal point. This is almost always supra-umbilical and usually central in position, although it may lie in either the right or left subcostal regions. It may be intermittent, periodic or persistent but the cardinal feature is that exacerbations are related in time to eating.

The cause is usually organic and the structures most frequently involved are the oesophagus, stomach, duodenum, gallbladder or pancreas.

2 Flatulent Indigestion

This less definite clinical variety is often accompanied by physical distension of the upper abdomen. Eructation is frequent but results in only temporary relief. It is less commonly indicative of organic disease in the stomach or duodenum and although inflammatory processes elsewhere in the abdominal cavity may be responsible, anxiety is a frequent cause.

Aerophagy is an exaggerated form of flatulence in which air is swallowed, temporarily stored in the oesophagus and intermittently released with dramatic effect and the claim of considerable relief.

3 Regurgitant Indigestion

This is described by patients as heartburn or acidity and results from the contact of gastric juice with the oesophageal mucosa. While an hiatus hernia may occasionally be present, in the great majority of cases there is no such anatomical abnormality. If the regurgitation is persistently repeated an oesophagitis occurs, which in turn plays its part in perpetuating the situation.

4 Nauseous Indigestion

This is the commonest variety and has the widest range of causes. The following brief classification gives an indication of some of these:

(a) Infective
  (i) almost any febrile illness
  (ii) mild food poisoning
  (iii) hepatitis
(b) Congestive
  (i) heart failure
  (ii) alcohol—acute chronic

(c) Endocrine, Metabolic and Drugs
  (i) pregnancy
  (ii) thyrotoxicosis
  (iii) uraemia
  (iv) digitalis, etc
(d) Neurogenic
  (i) cerebral tumour
  (ii) migraine
  (iii) anxiety

It is helpful in these patients to determine whether the nausea is present continuously (uraemia), whether it occurs at the sight of food (hepatitis) or only after ingestion (i.e. aspirins and digitalis).

5 Anorexic Indigestion

This is a somewhat arbitrary distinction from nauseous indigestion of which it obviously forms an integral part but when the anorexia occurs alone, especially in older patients, carcinoma of the stomach should be suspected.

6 Exertional Indigestion

When a careful history is taken from a patient with coronary thrombosis, although he will frequently deny any preceding episodes of heart pain, he will often readily admit to experiencing 'indigestion'.

This symptom is true angina but it is misinterpreted by the patient as indigestion. The mechanism causing the pain is the increased demand placed on the myocardium due to the splanchnic vaso-dilatation after meals.

DIFFERENTIAL DIAGNOSIS

History is all important and provided it is given in detail and is sufficiently accurate, the majority of cases can be correctly diagnosed by this means alone. Particular note should be made of the following points:

1. The character of the discomfort and its timing.
2. The total duration and whether intermittent, periodic or persistent.

Indigestion

3 The time relationship to food and degree of response to antacid medication.
4 The preservation or loss of appetite.
5 The association with nausea or vomiting.
6 The presence of any associated symptoms.

INVESTIGATIONS

If organic disease is suspected, a Barium meal and follow-through, cholecystogram, gastroscopy and pancreatic studies may each or all be required depending on the initial diagnosis. A positive result is helpful but it must be recognised that negative results by no means exclude organic disease. In only two-thirds of proven cases of peptic ulcer can the lesion be demonstrated radiographically; gallstones are not always easy to demonstrate and the diagnosis of pancreatic disorders is notoriously difficult. In these patients a haemoglobin, white count, sedimentation rate and stool examination for parasites and occult blood may indicate that further investigations should be pursued.

NERVOUS DYSPEPSIA

Every day domestic and environmental stresses cause many people in whom there is no organic disease to complain of indigestion and it is important that the presence of this common condition should be deduced from direct evidence and a careful history and not diagnosed by exclusion after prolonged investigations. The implication of intensive search is that some serious disease may be present and this fear only intensifies anxiety, making management even more difficult. Nevertheless there are patients who need the supportive evidence of a normal X-ray (i.e. Barium meal) in addition to their doctor's reassurance to allay their fears and in these patients limited investigations can be both diagnostic and therapeutic.

CHAPTER 4

PEPTIC ULCER

Peptic ulcers are always associated with the presence of gastric mucosal secretion. They can therefore only occur in the:
> **Oesophagus (the lower end)**
> **Hiatus hernia**
> **Stomach**
> **Duodenum (the first part)**
> **Duodenum and jejunum in the Zollinger-Ellison syndrome**
> **Jejunum following gastro-enterostomy**
> **Meckel's diverticulum**

Classification
> 1 Acute
> 2 Subacute
> 3 Chronic

1 Acute peptic ulcer
These are often multiple but are normally shortlived. They occur as a result of minor dietary indiscretions but they are rarely of clinical importance since the majority heal rapidly and spontaneously.

Curling's ulcer which occurs in response to extensive burns and also Cushing's ulcer which may follow a mid-brain lesion are rarer examples of acute ulceration.

2 Subacute (recurrent) peptic ulcer
This is more frequently duodenal and is usually associated with an above average gastric secretory output. The main problem in such cases is the prevention of recurrences since spontaneous healing will occur.

3 Chronic (persistent) peptic ulcer

These ulcers may be either gastric or duodenal but the causative factors are probably different in the two circumstances.

There is a great variety in their form which may be large or small, shallow or deep. In the active stage the ulcer gives rise to symptoms of indigestion and pain and even in the quiescent stage of fibrosis, complications of stenosis and adherence to other viscera may occur.

Aetiology

There is no single factor responsible for peptic ulceration since it is a specialised form of injury and not a specific disease.

1. Acid secretion. In general duodenal ulcer is related to hypersecretion whereas gastric ulcer is more often associated with nutritional factors but in neither case is this invariable.
2. Sex and age. Duodenal ulcer occurs with greatest frequency in early middle age and in males whereas gastric ulcer has its highest incidence in later life with a predominance of females.
3. Heredity. Heredity plays a part in some cases of duodenal ulcers and affected families can usually be shown to be hypersecretors of acid.
4. Stress. Anxiety, worry and strain provoke hypersecretion via the vagal pathways. These conditions are therefore more likely to result in duodenal rather than gastric ulceration.
5. Diet. The effects of diet are not clearly defined but the current custom of taking tea, coffee, alcohol and nicotine on an empty stomach may be significant as these all stimulate gastric secretion.

Clinical features

1. Periodicity of symptoms is the most reliable feature and this is evidence of the natural history of the condition, i.e. periodic relapse with spontaneous healing.
2. A constant time relation between the symptoms and the taking of food is important but is not specific in the differentiation of gastric from duodenal ulcers.

3 Relief with antacids, especially if transient, is suggestive of peptic ulceration but it should be recognised that these agents benefit most forms of dyspepsia.
4 Pain is most frequently high in the epigastric angle rather than over the anatomical site of the ulcer. It can vary in position but is always above the umbilicus. Occasionally discomfort may be retrosternal and is due to oesophageal reflux or spasm.

   Night pain is suggestive of duodenal ulcer but sleep is not necessarily disturbed even in long-standing cases.

   Back pain usually means adherence to and penetration of posterior abdominal wall structures, especially the pancreas. Unremitting pain often has the same significance.
5 Appetite as such is retained although the patient may avoid food because of the fear of experiencing pain.
6 Nausea and vomiting may occur with severe pain but are not persistent except as a result of complications.

Complications

These may be:

1 Haemorrhage

Bleeding may be
  (1) sudden and severe and give rise to haematemesis and melaena or
  (ii) less severe and chronic giving rise to symptoms of anaemia. Blood loss may only be detected in the faeces by chemical means.

2 Perforation

This may occur into the general peritoneal cavity or into the lesser sac. There may be little previous history of indigestion.

3 Penetration

Peptic ulcers may adhere to and involve the liver or pancreas.

4 Stenosis

Fibrosis associated with high gastric ulcers may result in an hourglass deformity of the stomach. When associated with pyloric

Peptic Ulcer

or duodenal ulcers it will result in outflow obstruction and gastric distension (pyloric stenosis).

5 Carcinoma

Probably in only a very few instances does cancer arise in a previously benign gastric ulcer although carcinomas may themselves ulcerate.

Malignant change does not occur in duodenal ulcers.

Investigations

1. Barium meal X-rays.

   The majority (80%) of ulcers can be seen on a Barium meal but posterior gastric and duodenal ulcers may be difficult to demonstrate. A patient with a negative X-ray result in the presence of symptoms should be kept under review.

2. Gastric function tests.

   A high acid output supports a diagnosis of duodenal ulcer and achlorhydria excludes benign peptic ulceration but function tests are never diagnostic.

3. Gastroscopy.

   This should be considered complementary to radiography and is particularly useful in demonstrating acute ulcers which may not be detected by X-rays. Fibre-optic instruments have made gastroscopy easier and more practicable particularly for the elderly. High gastric lesions are difficult to see with any of the instruments currently available.

Treatment

Medical Management.

It is important that the patient should recognise and accept responsibility for his progress since medicine alone will never cure an ulcer although it may considerably relieve symptoms. Only overall readjustments by the patient himself can ensure complete success.

1 Diet

It is convenient to have a printed schedule of instructions available but these while being decisive should be permissive rather than restrictive.

(a) Meals should be small, frequent and regular so using the natural buffering action of foods. Meals should be two-hourly at first but later a 'between meal feeding' plan is adequate. This is more easily understood than advising 'something to eat every three hours'.

(b) The constitution of the diet is less important than regular meals but in the early stages the diet should be bland. Nicotine and alcohol should be denied in the early weeks although some latitude may be allowed later. Neither should be taken on an empty stomach. The same instructions should apply to very hot or cold drinks, spices, onions and gaseous drinks.

2 Drugs

(a) Antacid preparations.

Total neutralisation of gastric acid is impossible but fortunately to control symptoms it is sufficient to neutralise the *excess* acid production. Treatment should be continuous with frequent small doses. In the early stages alternate food and medicine at hourly intervals may be necessary but later a less intensive régime is acceptable.

Although food buffers acid, a meal stimulates acid secretion and symptoms usually occur after food. Antacids should therefore be given between meals but before the usual time of occurrence of the patient's pain.

Liquid antacids are usually more effective than tablets but many patients who have to travel during the course of their work find tablets more practicable.

Choice of the large range of Magnesium, Aluminium and Calcium salts is largely empirical but not all these compounds are non-absorbable and therefore free of the danger of alkalosis or, in the case of calcium carbonate, hypercalcaemia.

(b) Anticholinergics

These agents act
  (i) by vagal blockade thus exerting some control over excess acid production
  (ii) as antispasmodics, reducing gastro-duodenal muscular tone and thus relieving pain.

Pure atropine alkaloid or tincture of belladonna given three or four times a day are still widely employed and it is doubtful if synthetic preparations are superior although some patients respond better to one than to another.

In the relief of pain they should be given if necessary in increasing doses to the limit of tolerance of side effects (i.e. dry mouth, impairment of visual accommodation, dysuria etc.)

(c) Sedatives

Although there is no evidence that the use of these accelerate the healing of ulcers they are of undoubted symptomatic value and by reducing emotional tension they diminish acid output.

In order to avoid fatigue and depression the short acting varieties are preferable for use during the day (amytal 30-45 mgms. three times a day) with an additional dose to cover any extra emotional stress. At night meprobamate 400 mgms. is a useful preparation.

(d) Carbenoxolone sodium (Biogastrone)

This compound isolated from liquorice extract has been shown to accelerate the healing of gastric ulcers in ambulant patients in a dosage of 100 mgms. three times a day. It appears to have a local action on the gastric mucosa the exact nature of which is uncertain.

Unfortunately there is a liability to fluid and sodium retention and for these reasons the drug should not be used in cases of hypertension or heart disease.

3 Preventative long-term measures

Since healing of peptic ulcers is spontaneous but recurrence so frequent. prophylaxis might well be considered to be more important than initial therapy.

As soon as any individual attack is controlled relaxation of the dietetic and medicinal régime is permissible but patients should maintain the habit of taking meal supplements or of sucking an antacid tablet at these interval times in lieu of food.

There should be a brief return to the full régime before or following any particular circumstance or event liable to provoke a relapse.

Surgical management

Surgical treatment may be indicated in cases of:
(i) profuse haemorrhage, not quickly controlled by medical measures
(ii) recurrent haemorrhage
(iii) other complications—i.e. perforation pyloric stenosis
(iv) failure of gastric ulcers to heal on medical treatment
(v) Inability to keep at full-time work due to recurrent symptoms from duodenal ulceration.

Procedures in current practice are:

1 Gastro-enterostomy.
   This diverts the acid flow away from the ulcer but does not modify the subsequent acid secretion and in consequence there is a high recurrence rate. It is a valuable procedure in the elderly or poor risk patient who can be shown to have only a moderate acid output.

2 Partial gastrectomy
   (a) Bilroth I—stomach remnant anastomosed direct to divided second part of duodenum. Direct continuity.
   (b) Polya—stomach remnant anastomosed to loop of jejunum. Proximal duodenum closed. Altered flow.
   Both operations are designed to remove part of the ulcer bearing area of the stomach and at the same time reduce the hormonal (gastrin) influence on gastric secretion.

3 Vagotomy and pyloroplasty.
   Vagotomy will reduce acid secretion but carried out by itself leads to gastric retention. It is therefore always combined with a drainage procedure, either pyloroplasty or gastro-enterostomy.

Post-operative complications

Apart from the immediate problem of haemorrhage or sepsis there are several sequelae which can give rise to considerable difficulty in management.

1 Short term complications

These usually occur within weeks or months of the operation and on occasions may settle spontaneously. Further surgery is

avoided where possible.
- (a) Bilious vomiting—sometimes called the 'afferent loop syndrome—may follow a Polya gastrectomy. It is due to pooling of biliary and pancreatic secretions in the closed off duodenal loop—these are vomited ½ to 1 hour after taking food. The diagnostic feature is the absence of food in the vomit which may be of considerable volume.
- (b) The so called 'dumping syndrome' is less frequently encountered and its full explanation is not yet known. Too rapid filling of the jejunum, over-distension of the efferent loop, reactive hypoglycaemia, electrolyte disturbance and tension of the stomach remnant on its retroperitoneal attachment have all been incriminated.

    Symptoms consist of sense of faintness, sweating, tachycardia and a feeling of distension after meals. Relief is usually obtained from lying flat immediately after taking food.
- (c) Diarrhoea may prove a serious problem after vagotomy operations although the majority of patients are merely relieved of the pre-existing state of constipation.

    Selective vagotomy has been claimed to prevent this complication but this is still a controversial point.

2 Long term complications

These occur after a period of years and the longer the follow-up, the higher is the incidence of complications. They result from a combination of poor intake, rapid transit and diversion or alteration of the normal flow of gastric contents and biliary and pancreatic secretions.
- (a) Weight loss may be a problem, especially in instances of high gastrectomy and can only be countered by increased intake.
- (b) Anaemia is a complication and should be anticipated by routine administration of haematinics. It is most commonly of iron deficiency type but a macrocytic anaemia may follow vitamin B_{12} or folic acid insuffiiency.
- (c) Bone disease, either osteoporosis or even osteomalacia may develop after the lapse of many years and is a further reason for keeping patients under permanent surveillance after gastric surgery.

CHAPTER 5

ACUTE GASTRO-INTESTINAL BLEEDING

Haematemesis and melaena
Frank rectal bleeding

HAEMATEMESIS AND MELAENA

The commonest causes are:
  Acute gastric erosion
  Peptic ulcer
  Hiatus hernia
  Oesophageal varices
  Carcinoma of the stomach

Other causes are numerous and include benign tumours of the stomach, telangiectatic vessels and anti-coagulant therapy.

It should be remembered that in 10—15% of even the severe cases the source of bleeding cannot be demonstrated.

Clinical features
1 There will be evidence of unaltered bright red blood or altered brown (coffee grounds) blood in the vomit.
2 Most cases of haematemesis will subsequently have black tarry (melaena) stools.
3 All will subsequently have stools chemically positive for blood.
4 In severe cases the pulse will be rapid, the patient will be pale and sweating and may later become shocked. Note: A

Acute Gastro-intestinal Bleeding

litre or more of blood can be lost before symptoms become obvious and the patient's condition may worsen suddenly when the blood volume drops below a critical level.

Diagnosis of source

(a) Past history:
  (i) has there been any previous indigestion ?
  (ii) has there been a high alcohol intake ?
  (iii) has the patient been taking drugs i.e. aspirin, butazolidin, steroids ?

(b) Clinical examination:
  Look for (i) stigmata of liver disease
  (ii) tenderness in the abdomen (in some cases of peptic ulceration)
  (iii) mass in the epigastrium (in some cases of carcinoma)
  (iv) bruising on the skin (in blood disorders)
  (v) telangiectasia in the skin (in hereditary telangiectasia).

Investigations

1. Haemoglobin. Initially may be high before haemodilution occurs but later falls. Serial haemoglobin estimates are therefore important.
2. Differential white count and film may show blood dyscrasia i.e. leukaemia.
3. Prothrombin time may be abnormal in liver disease or during anticoagulant therapy.
4. Plain X-ray of chest may show large hiatus hernia.
5. Limited Barium meal (i) after washing out the stomach or (ii) within 48 hours of cessation of bleeding may reveal the presence of gross lesions without precipitating further bleeding and help in immediate management.
6. Detailed Barium studies can be made when the urgent situation is past.
7. Endoscopy, particularly with a fibrescope, can be carried out early—in the ward if necessary—and may reveal acute erosions that will not be detected later.

FRANK RECTAL BLEEDING

The commonest causes are:
>   **Haemorrhoids**
>   **Carcinoma of rectum and colon**
>   **Ulcerative colitis**
>   **Diverticulitis**

Other causes include ischaemic infarction, Crohn's disease and other tumours of the colon.

Clinical features

1 Blood from lesions in the sigmoid and rectum is usually bright red but from proximal colonic lesions will be darker in colour unless the bleeding is profuse.
2 In severe cases the patient may become shocked from blood loss alone but in cases where there is associated fluid loss due to diarrhoea, a state of collapse may occur earlier.

Diagnosis of source

(a) Past history:
  (i) has there been any change in bowel habit?
  (ii) is there associated diarrhoea of the passage of mucus?
  (iii) has there been abdominal pain?
(b) Clinical examination:
  Look for (i) presence of prolapsed haemorrhoids
  (ii) evidence of an abdominal mass (in cases of carcinoma or diverticulitis)
  (iii) presence of abdominal tenderness (in cases of diverticulitis)
  (iv) presence of abdominal distension due to faeces or flatus proximal to obstruction by carcinoma or stasis due to ulcerative colitis.

Investigations

1 Digital rectal examination and proctoscopy should be carried out in all cases and will demonstrate haemorrhoids and low rectal tumours.
2 Sigmoidoscopy should be carried out in all cases and will

Acute Gastro-intestinal Bleeding

demonstrate higher rectal tumours and inflammatory or ulcerative rectal disease.
3 A plain X-ray of the abdomen may show colonic distension, faecal stasis and in some cases of ulcerative colitis mucosal irregularity.
4 An 'instant' Barium enema without prior preparation may be helpful in diagnosing gross disease.
5 A Barium enema with double contrast radiography will demonstrate the majority of colonic lesions and can be carried out after the urgent situation is past.

Treatment of gastro-intestinal bleeding

All cases, no matter how mild they may at first appear, should be treated as serious.

General management
1 An accurate fluid intake and output record must be kept and an assessment made of the blood content of vomit and faeces before and after admission.
2 Determination of the patient's blood group and the organisation of an adequate supply of suitable blood is an immediate responsibility.
3 If the history suggests the loss of a litre or more of blood then early transfusion is indicated regardless of the recorded haemoglobin level. Should the haemoglobin level be 50% or lower, blood replacement is essential and urgent.
4 Clinical observation of pulse and blood pressure should be frequent—$\frac{1}{4}$ or $\frac{1}{2}$ hourly initially. A rising pulse and falling blood pressure are ominous and are indications for immediate restoration of blood volume.
5 Blood replacement requirements can be more accurately assessed by measuring the central venous pressure through an indwelling catheter. This technique gives early warning of further blood loss and its use can prevent over transfusion.
6 Sedation is necessary to allay anxiety and lessen shock. Morphia tends to provoke vomiting and if used is preferably given with an antihistamine or anti-emetic drug.

Care must be taken when using opiates in cases of haemorrhage due to cirrhosis for fear of precipitating coma.

Surgery

The problem of whether or when to operate depends on
  (i) the diagnosis
  (ii) the age of the patient
  (iii) the general condition of the patient
and a consultation between the physician and surgeon should take place early in each case.
(a) Upper gastro-intestinal tract:
  It is impossible to lay down hard and fast rules but few would challenge the view that if haemorrhage recurs after resuscitation, then the patient should be retransfused and arrangements made to operate as soon as his condition is satisfactory.

  Early surgery is to be recommended in middle-aged or elderly patients since
  (i) they are more likely to be bleeding from an arteriosclerotic vessel in the base of a chronic ulcer.
  (ii) they are less able to withstand profound blood loss.
Surgery should be avoided if possible in the patients with acute ulcers or liver disease.

Blind laparotomy is occasionally necessary as a life-saving measure.

Gastric cooling has been used as a means of controlling haemorrhage but has not achieved popularity in this country.
(b) Rectal bleeding:
  Local injection or ligation of haemorrhoids may be necessary.

  Definitive surgery can usually be deferred until investigations are completed.

CHAPTER 6

THE LIVER

Classification of disorders:
1 **Virus infections**
    (a) **Infective hepatitis**
    (b) **Serum hepatitis**
    (c) **Glandular fever**
    (d) **Yellow fever**
2 **Spirochaetal infections**
    (a) **Leptospirosis**
    (b) **Syphilis**
3 **Bacterial infections**
    (a) **Acute**
        (i) **ascending cholangitis**
        (ii) **portal pyaemia**
    (b) **Chronic—tuberculosis**
4 **Infestations**
    (a) **Amoebiasis**
    (b) **Bilharziasis**
    (c) **Hydatid cysts**
5 **Poisons and drugs**
    (a) **'Hepato-toxins'—alcohol, carbon tetrachloride etc.**
    (b) **'Hepato-allergens'—chlorpromazine etc.**
6 **Cirrhosis**
    (a) **Portal (Laennec)**
    (b) **Post-viral (post-necrotic scarring)**
    (c) **Biliary**
7 **Tumours**
    (a) **Primary**
        (i) **benign**
        (ii) **malignant**

40   *Lecture Notes on Gastroenterology*

           (b) Secondary deposits
8 **Infiltrations**
           (a) The Reticuloses
           (b) The Leukaemias
           (c) The Lipoidoses
           (d) Amyloidosis
           (e) **Disseminated lupus erythematosus**
           (f) Sarcoidosis
9 **Metabolic Disorders**
           (a) Wilson's disease (copper)
           (b) Haemochromatosis (iron)
           (c) Porphyria (porphyrins)

1 VIRUS INFECTIONS

(a) Infective hepatitis

Aetiology

This is the most prevalent of all liver disorders in this country. Infection is contracted by ingestion of the virus and after reaching the intestine is spread via the blood stream. Although a contagious disease, infectivity is low and epidemics may occur in tightly crowded communities e.g. chronic hospitals and military camps. The incubation period is approximately three weeks and patients are likely to be infectious for at least ten days before jaundice appears as well as for a few days afterwards.

Pathology

Acute inflammatory changes occur throughout the liver and are characterized by centrilobular liver cell necrosis and an increased inflammatory cell infiltration particularly in the portal tracts. Polymorphonuclear cells, lymphocytes and plasma cells are found.

    In the majority of cases complete resolution occurs. Occasionally the destruction may be more severe and the condition then gradually progresses to a coarse type of cirrhosis known as post-necrotic scarring.

    Exceptionally infection may be so severe as to destroy all the parenchymal cells simultaneously (acute yellow atrophy) and

The Liver

in such cases death can occur even before the appearance of jaundice.

Clinical features

The majority of cases present as an acute illness and recover completely. The commonest features are:

1. A prodromal period of up to a week with general malaise, anorexia, nausea and a low grade fever.
2. Abdominal pain is uncommon but the patient may feel sore and tender over the liver.
3. Jaundice appears after the prodromal period and progressively deepens over a few days. It usually lasts two to three weeks but may be present for a few days only or last for several months. Jaundice tends to persist longer in the elderly.
4. The urine is dark in most patients due to bile pigments and the stools normal or slightly paler than normal. In some cases the obstructive element ('cholestatic jaundice') predominates and the stools become putty coloured.
5. Pruritis is unusual.
6. The liver may be palpable one or two fingers breadths below the costal margin but the edge is smooth and well defined. Splenomegaly may be found in one-fifth of cases.
7. There is a relative bradycardia and sometimes hypotension.

Other clinical presentations can be:

1. Subicteric hepatitis:
   In these cases, commonly children, although there are few symptoms and no jaundice, the patient feels unwell and may have a tender liver. Liver function tests may show a raised transaminase level and flocculation tests and a liver biopsy may reveal active hepatitis. Diagnosis is difficult but recovery is complete as far as is known.
2. Fulminating hepatitis:
   In exceptional instances the viral infection is severe enough to cause death with a week to ten days. Vomiting, drowsiness, coma and delirium occur in association with high fever, jaundice and widespread haemorrhages.
3. Relapsing hepatitis:
   Some cases present with an acute attack which appears to

recover but then recurs. There may be more than one relapse but recovery is complete.

4 Subacute hepatitis:
These patients present with an acute attack but this does not resolve completely. Jaundice persists or fluctuates, the patient feels ill and signs of liver failure develop within weeks. Mortality is high and although a few patients recover, they develop cirrhosis later.

5 Cirrhosis: (post-necrotic scarring)
Although rare, cirrhosis develops in a few patients after virus hepatitis. The scarring tends to be coarser than in 'portal cirrhosis'.

Investigations

1 Liver function tests.
   (a) The serum bilirubin level gives a quantitative measure of the jaundice.
   (b) The serum alkaline phosphatase is normal or slightly raised.
   (c) Flocculation reactions are abnormally high.
   (d) The serum transaminases are raised.
2 Percutaneous liver biopsy.
   This may show inflammatory changes.

Treatment

As is the case in most virus infections there is no specific therapy available but the following general measures should be adopted.

1 The patient should be kept at rest until the jaundice shows clear signs of remitting.
2 Diet should be normal and must contain adequate protein and glucose. At the onset of the desease there is almost always a definite distaste for fats but there is no need to restrict these later.
3 Alcohol should be avoided for six months.
4 Antibiotics and steroids do not significantly alter the course of the disease. Prednisolone (20 mgms. daily for five days) may be of help as a clinical test in the differentiation of cholestatic jaundice due to hepatitis from obstructive

The Liver

jaundice. Most cases of hepatitis show a transient lessening of jaundice.

(b) Serum hepatitis

Aetiology

This disorder is transmitted by means of infected serum and can occur as a result of using contaminated syringes for any type of injection, following blood transfusion or the use of pooled plasma. The incubation period is approximately three months.

Pathology
Clinical Features
Investigations
Treatment
} These are the same as in infective hepatitis. The mortality however is higher in serum hepatitis.

(c) Glandular fever (infectious mononucleosis)

Aetiology

The glandular fever virus affects the reticulo-endothelial system generally and may cause hepatitis sometimes with jaundice.

Pathology

There is an inflammatory reaction in the liver with an increase in mononuclear cells in the sinusoids and portal tracts.

Clinical features

1. There will be general malaise and other systemic features such as lymphadenopathy, sore throat, etc.
2. The liver may be slightly enlarged and tender.
3. Jaundice is not uncommon.

Investigations

1. Liver function tests.
   These indicate parenchymal damage as in infective hepatitis with raised flocculation tests and a normal alkaline phosphatase. The bilirubin may be slightly raised.
2. Percutaneous liver biopsy.

This is rarely necessary but will show acute inflammatory changes.

Treatment

This consists of symptomatic measures with bed rest and light diet.

(d) Yellow fever

Aetiology

This highly lethal viral infection is transmitted by the Aedes Aegypti mosquito and occurs principally in South America and Africa.

Pathology

There is a diffuse necrosis of the parenchymal cells in the midzones of the lobules. Intranuclear inclusion bodies may be seen within the liver cells. Although necrosis may be severe, cirrhosis does not occur subsequently.

Clinical features

1. The incubation period is short, from 3—6 days, the patients then rapidly developing severe toxaemia with fever, vomiting and haemorrhagic jaundice.
2. Death may occur within nine days but if not, recovery begins within this time and is complete.

Investigations

1. The virus can be demonstrated by injecting serum taken within the first three days of the illness into mice and producing encephalitis.
2. Acute and convalescent sera will demonstrate a rising titre of antibodies.

Treatment

No specific drug is available but almost complete protection is afforded by inoculation with dried attenuated yellow fever vaccine.

2 SPIROCHAETAL INFECTIONS

(a) Leptospirosis (Weil's disease)

Aetiology

This disorder may be due to Leptospira icterohaemorrhagiae excreted from the kidneys of rats or to L. canicola found in dogs. Leptospira gain entry by being ingested or through an abrasion in the skin. Those who work in association with stagnant water, e.g. agricultural workers, sewer workers etc. are most exposed to infection.

Pathology

1 The liver changes are those of a periportal inflammatory infiltration with only slight cell necrosis.
2 Jaundice is partly due to liver damage and partly due to tissue haemorrhage.
3 Haemorrhage is largely due to capillary damage and thrombocytopaenia rather than hypoprothrombinaemia.

Clinical features

The incubation period is approximately 7—14 days and the clinical illness then has a sudden onset.

1 In the first week the spirochaete circulates in the blood and gives rise to fever, rigors, muscle pains and nausea. There may also be signs of cerebral irritation, pneumonitis and jaundice.
2 In the second week there is evidence of increasing renal, cardiac and hepatic damage and death may occur from **renal failure.**

Investigations

1 A white cell count shows a leucocytosis of 10,000—30,000.
2 The organism may be demonstrated in blood and C.S.F. in the first week and in the urine soon after.
3 A specific agglutination reaction will become positive after the second week.
4 Albuminuria is marked as the kidney is also severely affected.

5 Conjunctival congestion is common and the heart and voluntary muscles may also be involved.

Treatment
1 General supportive measures are required as this can be a severe illness.
2 Fluids should be plentiful because of the fever but a detailed chart must be kept of the urinary output.
3 Broad-spectrum antibiotics are usually given but their specificity for the leptospira in man is doubtful.

(b) Syphilis

Aetiology
This infection caused by the spirochaete Treponema pallidum is now not common but may affect the liver.

Pathology
1 In congenital syphilis the liver is infected with spirochaetes which reach it across the placenta. Diffuse hepatitis occurs and if untreated, will result in cirrhosis.
2 In the secondary stage, miliary granulomata can be found in the liver.
3 In the tertiary stage, gummata may be found in the liver and healing leads to very coarse scarring and lobulation (hepar lobatum).

Clinical features
1 Infants will be jaundiced, have liver enlargement and show other signs of congenital syphilis.
2 Jaundice and hepatic tenderness are present in the secondary stage.
3 Asymptomatic liver enlargement may be found in the tertiary stage.

Investigations
1 Liver biposy may confirm the diagnosis in congenital syphilis and demonstrate granulomata in the secondary stage.
2 Serological tests will confirm the diagnosis.

The Liver

Treatment

This is as for the systemic disease with penicillin intramuscularly.

3 BACTERIAL INFECTIONS

(a) Acute

  (i) Ascending cholangitis.

   In certain instances of gallbladder disease, especially in the presence of obstruction, bacteria may gain access to the liver by ascending the biliary channels.

   The condition is described more fully in the chapter of the Biliary Tract (Chapter 7).

  (ii) Portal Pyaemia.

Aetiology

The portal vein provides an alternative route by which bacteria can gain access to the liver. The commonest source of the infection is a septic thrombo-phlebitis associated with either appendicitis or diverticulitis but any suppurative process with portal vein drainage may be responsible.

Pathology

Portal pyaemia results in multiple intrahepatic abscesses, the right lobe of the liver being more heavily involved than the left. Solitary abscesses are rare.

Clinical features

1. Pyaemia is characterised by a high swinging fever, drenching sweats, rigors and severe toxaemia.
2. Local symptoms are often absent in the early stages but later there is pain and tenderness over an enlarged liver.
3. Shoulder pain may be referred from diaphragmatic irritation.

Investigations

1. Blood culture may be positive.
2. A white cell count shows polymorphonuclear leucocytosis.

Treatment

1 Intensive and prolonged antibiotic therapy.
2 Surgical drainage of the primary suppurative area wherever possible.

(b) Chronic

Tuberculosis

Granulomatous lesions may occur in the liver as a result of haematogenous spread of tubercle bacilli in the systemic disease. These usually resolve but may calcify and be demonstrated as focal lesions on plain X-ray.

4 INFESTATIONS

(a) Hepatic amoebiasis

Aetiology

Hepatic involvement occurs during the course of intestinal amoebiasis, the amoebae reaching the liver via the portal vein.

Pathology

The amoebae initially give rise to a focal hepatitis which consists of multiple microscopic abscesses. The large, solitary lesions seen in the later stages result from the coalescence of adjacent necrotic areas.

Clinical features

1 The stage of invasion is usually undetected.
2 The presence of a large abscess may give rise to:
    (a) Fever, rigors and malaise
    (b) Liver enlargement and tenderness. Pain may occur over the liver or be referred to the shoulder.
3 Chronic amoebic hepatitis can occur and be associated with nausea, anorexia and discomfort over the liver.

Investigations

1 A plain X-ray of the liver area may show elevation of the diaphragm.

The Liver

2 Radioisotopic scanning may demonstrate a filling defect.
3 Aspiration of the abscess in suspected cases after treatment has begun may confirm the diagnosis.
4 Sigmoidoscopy and stool examination may demonstrate intestinal amoebiasis.

Treatment

1 Emetine hydrochloride should be given in all cases. The dosage varies from three to six injections of 60 mgms. I.M. according to the severity. It is essential to take precautions against myocardial toxicity by means of complete bed rest and cardiac monitoring.
2 Chloroquin is also given and is particularly effective as it is concentrated over a hundredfold in the liver. The dosage is 250 mgms. q.d.s. Prolonged treatment (4—6 weeks) may be necessary to ensure eradication of the amoebae.

(b) Bilharziasis (hepatic schistosomiasis)

Aetiology

Schistosoma mansoni and japonicum are the two types most commonly affecting the liver. The organisms gain entry through the skin, reach the capillaries and are then spread widely. The liver is affected principally in cases of intestinal disease when ova reach it via the mesenteric veins.

Pathology

The ova block the intrahepatic branches of the portal system and give rise to local inflammatory reaction which results in progressive fibrosis, which may be fine or coarse, and later portal hypertension.

Clinical features

1 In the early stages of liver invasion there may be fever, local liver tenderness and enlargement and nausea.
2 In the later stages the liver becomes smaller and fibrotic and signs of portal hypertension with splenomegaly, ascites and varices may occur.

Investigations

1 Liver biopsy may confirm the diagnosis by demonstrating ova as well as the inflammatory reaction.
2 Stool and rectal examination may show evidence of rectal involvement.

Treatment

1 Chemotherapy with antimony compounds will reduce the number of adult worms.
2 Medical and surgical measures may be required for the treatment of portal hypertension.

(c) Hydatid cysts

Aetiology

Cysts occur in man as a result of the larval stage of infection with the tapeworm Taenia echinococcus. Dogs are the definitive hosts and man and sheep the intermediate hosts.

Pathology

The majority of cysts occur in the liver. They have a thick wall and may contain daughter cysts. Fluid from the cyst is thus able to cause further infestation if liberated as well as a violent allergic reaction.

Clinical features

1 Many cysts remain asymptomatic and are found by chance on X-ray due to calcification of their wall.
2 Liver enlargement and aching in the right upper quadrant may be caused by a large cyst.
3 Urticarial skin rashes may be present due to the allergic nature of the cyst fluid.
4 Shock may result from rupture of a cyst into the peritoneum.
5 There may be fever and rigors if the cyst becomes secondarily infected.

Investigations

1 A plain X-ray may show calcification in a cyst.

The Liver

2 A blood count may show eosinophilia.
3 The intradermal (Casoni) antigen test will be positive.
4 Specific complement fixation tests will be positive in three-quarters of cases.

Treatment

Asymptomatic calcified cysts may require no treatment but where possible in other cases surgical removal is indicated to prevent the anaphylactoid reactions of spontaneous rupture.

5 POISONS AND DRUGS

The liver cell is especially vulnerable to injury by chemical compounds. This is partly because it is actively concerned with the detoxication of many of them and partly because of the fact that it acts as a filter for the blood arriving direct from the intestinal absorption area.

Not only are a large number of compounds which are widely employed in industry potentially hazardous in this respect but in addition an ever increasing number of prescribed drugs are proving to have an adverse effect upon the liver.

Liver damage may be due to:

(a) The Hepato-toxins e.g. carbon tetrachloride
These cause damage to the parenchymal cells and in severe cases they may cause total destruction. The effect is directly proportional to the dosage.

(b) The Hepato-allergens e.g. chlorpromazine
these drugs cause a sensitivity reaction with intercellular oedema and obstruction of the biliary canaliculi ('cholestatic jaundice'). The effect is not proportional to the dosage.

In some cases the response by the liver is a mixture of the two types described.

A brief list of half a dozen of the more important members of each group is given below but it must be appreciated that the potential list is formidable.

Hepato-toxins	Hepato-allergens
Carbon tetrachloride	Chlorpromazine
Chloroform	Methyltestosterone
Ethyl alcohol	Phenylbutazone
Gold, antimony and arsenical compounds	Isonicotinic acid hydrazine
British anti lewisite	Tolbutamide and chlorpropamide
Amanita phalloides (mushrooms)	Phenindione

Clinical features

1. Jaundice occurs in both groups but systemic symptoms are more likely to occur with the toxins.
   The duration of the jaundice is unpredictable but in the case of drug reactions, cholestasis may be prolonged for many weeks.
2. There may be a prodromal period, extending from a few days to several weeks, during which the patient complains of non-specifice malaise, anorexia, nausea, vomiting and vague abdominal discomfort. This phase is virtually indistinguishable from the pre-icteric period of virus hepatitis.
3. The liver may be enlarged and exceedingly tender in the more acute instances of 'toxic' hepatitis. Splenomegaly is not a feature.
4. A careful search should be made for other evidence of tissue damage or allergy such as skin rashes, purpura, albuminuria and microscopic haematuria.
5. Meticulous cross-questioning of all cases of jaundice is imperative in order to discover any industrial or domiciliary risks and also the details of all previous medication.

Treatment

1. The toxic agent should be immediately withdrawn, hence the importance of establishing its identity as early as possible.
2. General measures consist of bed rest, free fluids and full, but not excessive, diet with adequate glucose.
3. Steroids. There is no convincing evidence that these are

beneficial in the treatment of the hepatitis although they may be useful in a short course in the differential diagnosis of obstructive jaundice (see page 42).

6 CIRRHOSIS

Cirrhosis has come to mean the process of healing with nodular regeneration and scarring occurring as a result of previous hepato-cellular injury.

(a) Portal cirrhosis

Aetiology

This is far the most common variety and may be associated with:

(i) excessive alcohol intake
(ii) malnutrition protein deficiency, Kwashiorkor
(iii) cardiac failure
(iv) schistosomiasis—Bilharzial infestation
(v) haemochromatosis—iron intoxication
(vi) Wilson's disease—copper intoxication
(vii) Syphilis
(viii) idiopathic—of undiscovered aetiology.

This last heading is included, since in addition to the first seven well recognised causes, there are almost certainly many others as yet undisclosed. In fact the majority of cases of cirrhosis in the younger age group in this country do not have any convincing aetiological explanation.

Pathology

Following liver injury due to the causes mentioned above there is first of all cell necrosis followed by collapse of the reticulin framework and an increase in fibrous tissue. As the damage is diffuse throughout the liver, fibrous bands form which disturb the normal architecture. Where cells have not been destroyed, nodules of regeneration develop and it is the combination of fibrosis and regeneration which gives rise to the fine nodularity of the liver surface.

In association with the fibrosis there is an increased cellular infiltration in the portal tracts as well as some proliferation of small bile ducts.

Clinical features

Scarring develops very gradually over a number of years and during this period cirrhosis gives no clinical indication of its presence.

When symptoms and signs appear they are due:
1. To interference with intrahepatic blood flow causing portal hypertension, the features of which are:
   (a) An enlarged firm finely nodular liver which later becomes impalpable due to contraction.
   (b) Splenomegaly.
   (c) Haematemesis and melaena from rupture of enlarged porto-systemic collateral veins in the oesophagus and stomach.
2. To hepatic insufficiency as a result of hepatocellular failure the features of which are:
   (a) Jaundice which when present is usually of mild to moderate degree and due to impaired conjugation and excretion.
   (b) Ascites and generalised oedema due to lowered serum albumen as a result of impaired liver synthesis.
   (c) Easy bruising due to altered prothrombin levels.
   (d) Spider naevi which may be seen over the upper part of the body, 'liver palms' with reddening of the thenar and hypothenar eminences and gynaecomastia, all possibly associated with disturbed oestrogen metabolism.
   (e) Disordered behaviour, a curious flapping tremor of outstretched hands and finally coma and death due to neurological damage.

Investigations
1. Liver function tests will help in the assessment of parenchymal damage and the presence of activity of the disease process. Extensive cirrhotic changes can occur without much derangement of liver function tests.
2. Serum proteins may indicate low albumen levels.

The Liver

3 Blood count may show anaemia.
4 Prothrombin times may be prolonged.
5 Liver biopsy will confirm changes of cirrhosis.
6 Barium swallow may show oesophageal varices.
7 A splenic venogram will demonstrate the collateral circulation and the portal pressure can be measured at the same time.
8 Radioisotopic scanning may be helpful in demonstrating a coarse pattern.
9 An E.E.G. may show changes in cases of hepatic precoma.

Treatment

1 Complete withdrawal of alcohol is obligatory even when this is not the aetiological agent.
2 A nutritious diet should be provided with particular emphasis upon adequate proteins, calories and vitamins. Supplemental vitamin B is traditional in alcoholic cirrhosis but is almost certainly beneficial in all types. A high protein intake is particularly necessary in the presence of either oedema or ascites (except where there is precoma) since these denote low serum albumen levels.
3 Diuretics are also of use in cases with ascites. A particularly valuable combination is Hydrochlorothiazide 50 mgms. and Spironolactone (an aldosterone antagonist) 25 mgms. given once, twice or three times a day.
4 The treatment of oesophageal varices is considered separately in Chapter 1.

Hepatic pre-coma or coma

Aetiology

This is the result of severe liver failure and is often precipitated by some additional event such as a massive gastro-intestinal haemorrhage from oesophageal varices, an intercurrent infection, abdominal paracentesis, narcotic medication or even a large protein meal.

Pathology

Due to impaired liver function and shunting of portal blood

into the systemic circulation, the nervous system is exposed to high levels of blood ammonia and other toxins (portal systemic encephalopathy).

Clinical features

The patient becomes confused, at times quite suddenly, is ataxic and has a flapping tremor of the hands. Coma and death follow if untreated.

Investigations
1. Blood ammonia levels may be raised.
2. An E.E.G. may show an abnormal pattern.

Treatment
1. Protein should be withdrawn altogether but the total calorie intake should be maintained as near to 1500-2000 calories as possible by means of carbohydrate alone.
2. Purging with magnesium sulphate is used to eliminate protein from the lumen of the alimentary tract. This is especially relevant where there has been an intra-intestinal bleed. Rectal washouts are also valuable.
3. The administration of Neomycin 4—6 gm. for four to five days further benefits by reducing bacterial activity in the bowel. Milk protein diets may also be of value in the short term management. In cases persistently on the verge of coma, long term Neomycin may be necessary.

(b) Post-viral hepatitis (post-necrotic scarring)

This variety of cirrhosis can follow severe viral hepatitis and is only differentiated from portal cirrhosis by the fact that the scarring is coarse rather than fine.

(c) Biliary cirrhosis

Aetiology

This results from prolonged obstructive jaundice which may be due to:
1. A primary disorder of unknown aetiology associated with chronic intrahepatic obstruction and cholestasis.

The Liver

2 Extrahepatic obstruction with or without ascending biliary infection.

Pathology

The liver is enlarged, dark green and finely nodular. There is an increase in the number of bile ducts, the biliary canaliculi are distended and bile lakes and bile thrombi can be seen. In the portal tracts there is mononuclear cell infiltration and progressive fibrosis. Nodular regeneration occurs and the picture of cirrhosis develops.

Clinical features

1 Jaundice is invariable and deep. The patient's colour becomes greenish rather than yellow.
2 Pruritus is common.
3 Xanthomata may be seen on the eyelids, hands, buttocks and over joints and pressure areas.
4 The liver is enlarged and firm.
5 Steatorrhoea occurs due to interruption of the enterohepatic circulation of bile salts.

Investigations

1 The serum bilirubin and alkaline phosphatase are raised.
2 The serum lipids and cholesterol are increased.
3 Liver biopsy will show the changes of biliary cirrhosis.
4 Plain X-ray and a Barium meal may demonstrate a cause of extrahepatic obstruction.
5 Percutaneous cholangiography may help in determining the site of obstruction.

Treatment

1 Surgery is indicated wherever possible in cases of extrahepatic obstruction.
2 For primary biliary cirrhosis there is no specific treatment and symptomatic measures should include:
   (a) Alleviation of pruritus with local skin applications and cholestyramine or androgens if necessary.
   (b) Replacements of fat soluble vitamins and calcium lost due to steatorrhoea.

7 TUMOURS

(a) Primary

(i) Benign.
These are rare and almost all cell types within the liver have been recorded as forming a tumour e.g. angioma, fibroma etc.

(ii) Malignant.

Aetiology

A primary cancer of the liver is surprisingly uncommon in spite of the frequent occurrence of cirrhosis. In about two-thirds of all cases of primary cancer there is an associated cirrhosis and yet in certain African communities who neither take alcohol nor have any significant incidence of cirrhosis, there is a high incidence of liver cancer.

Haemochromatosis and Bilharziasis are also associated with a higher incidence of malignant change.

Pathology

The tumour may develop from the parenchymal cells (hepatoma) or bile ducts (cholangioma). More rarely sarcomas of various cell types are encountered.

Clinical features

1. General malaise and weight loss dominate the picture but symptoms are understandably variable and the onset is always indeterminate.
2. Gross hepatomegaly may develop and pain may be considerable.
3. In the terminal phase hypoglycaemic episodes may precede the more usual features of hepatic failure.

Investigations

1. Liver biopsy may enable the primary nature of the tumour to be indentified.
2. Radioisotopic scanning may define the limits of the tumour.

Treatment

This is usually palliative but the following should be considered:
1. Partial hepatectomy
2. Chemotherapy
3. Regional perfusion

(b) Secondary deposits

Aetiology

These are as common as the foregoing are rare and almost all cancers eventually seed themselves in the liver. As might be expected those growths located in the territory of the portal vein metastasise most freely such as tumours of the stomach, colon and pancreas.

Clinical features

Symptoms are few and the majority of patients succumb from hepatic coma without undue distress.

Investigations

1. Liver biopsy. This may be successful in demonstrating malignant deposits.
2. Radioisotopic scanning may show a clear area in the liver.

Treatment

The relative lack of symptoms provides justification for radical excision of a primary symptomatic malignant lesion when practicable even if hepatic secondaries are already present at the time of operation.

8 INFILTRATIONS

(a) The reticuloses

At autopsy over two-thirds of patients succumbing to Hodgkin's disease are found to have liver involvement. This is less frequently apparent clinically but when obvious it is of ominous significance.

Jaundice does not necessarily indicate hepatic infiltration since this symptom is sometimes due to pressure of enlarged glands in the porta hepatis.

(b) The leukaemias

The liver is involved in some degree in almost all types of leukaemia but gross enlargement usually indicates chronic myeloid leukaemia.

Multiple myeloma and polycythaemia vera rubra may also produce hepatomegaly.

(c) The lipoidoses

These comprise a group of conditions, most of which have a familial basis, in which there is a disorder of lipid metabolism. There is an accumulation of the intermediate products in the reticulo-endothelial cells which give rise to hepato-splenomegaly.

The group comprises Gaucher's disease, Neimann-Pick disease, varous xanthomatoses and possibly even eosinophilic granuloma.

(d) Amyloidosis

The liver may become infiltrated with amyloid in chronic diseases such as tuberculosis, lung abscess or rheumatoid arthritis (secondary amyloidosis) or less commonly in primary amyloidosis. The smooth liver enlargement is usually asymptomatic and treatment is for the causative condition.

(e) Systemic lupus erythematosus

Lupoid hepatitis is one facet of the ill-defined disorder associated with the appearance of L.E. cells in the peripheral blood. The liver enlargement is due more to an inflammatory reaction than true infiltration.

(f) Sarcoidosis

In this disorder of unknown aetiology granulomatous lesions may be found diffusely scattered throughout the liver in two-thirds of patients. Liver biopsy will confirm their presence and is used as a means of confirming the diagnosis suspected on other grounds.

The Liver

9 METABOLIC DISORDERS

(a) Wilson's disease (hepatolenticular degeneration)

Aetiology

This is a rare disorder of copper metabolism associated with a deficiency of the α_2 globulin required for copper transfer in the plasma (caeruloplasmin).

Pathology

Copper absorption from the intestine is increased and excessive amounts are deposited in the tissues. In the liver this leads to a coarse post-necrotic type of cirrhosis and in the brain to degeneration of the basal ganglia.

Clinical features

Patients commonly present in adolescence with:
1. Enlargement of the liver and ascites and haematemesis due to portal hypertension.
2. Dystonia, tremor, rigidity and pseudo-bulbar symptoms due to neurological involvement.
3. Greenish pigmentation at the periphery of the cornea due to mineral deposits (Kayser-Fleischer rings).

Investigations

1. Liver biopsy will confirm the presence of excess copper and cirrhosis.
2. Blood levels of caeruloplasmin are usually raised.

Treatment

Penicillamine hydrochloride, a chelating agent, should be given by mouth to increase urinary copper excretion.

(b) Haemochromatosis

Aetiology

This is a rare disorder of iron metabolism in which there is an excessive absorption of iron from the intestine. It is a familial disorder in which relatives of patients with clinical haemochromatosis are frequently found to have abnormal serum iron levels.

Pathology

Increased intestinal absorption leads to deposition of large quantities of iron in the tissues generally but it is particularly marked in the liver and pancreas. In the liver the iron gives rise to a chronic fibrous reaction and leads to cirrhosis. In the pancreas iron deposition leads to diabetes mellitus.

Clinical features

The damaging effect or iron in the different organs causes their eventual failure and the commonest features are:
1. Brown or slate grey pigmentation of the skin
2. An enlarged liver and later signs of cirrhosis
3. Diabetes mellitus
4. Adrenal and testicular insufficiency
5. Heart failure

Investigations
1. Serum iron levels will be raised and the unsaturated iron binding capacity will be reduced.
2. Liver biopsy will confirm both the excessive iron deposit and the cirrhosis.
3. A glucose tolerance curve may confirm the presence of diabetes.

Treatment
1. Venesection (phlebotomy) of 500 ml weekly over a period of approximately two years will reduce iron stores. Less frequent venesection may be required subsequently.
2. The Chelating agent desferrioxamine may be used to increase urinary excretion of iron. This method is slower and less effective than venesection.
3. Hormonal treatment, i.e. insulin, testosterone, etc., may be needed to treat endocrine deficiencies.

(c) Porphyria

Aetiology

An excess of circulating porphyrins occurs as a result of hepatic dysfunction. This may be due to a genetic disorder (porphyria hepatica) or be secondary to chronic alcoholism or chemical poisons.

Clinical features

These are due to the circulating porphyrins and are:
1. Photosensitivity
2. Abdominal colic
3. Peripheral neuritis
4. Psychiatric disorders

Investigations

1. Urinary porphyrins are increased.
2. Liver function tests and liver biopsy may be abnormal in secondary cases.

Treatment

There is no specific treatment for this disorder but obvious precipitating causes, such as alcohol and drugs (particularly barbiturates), should be avoided.

CHAPTER 7

THE BILIARY TRACT

The following are the conditions most frequently encountered in the biliary tract:
        Congenital anomalies
        Cholelithiasis (stones)
        Infection: Cholecystitis—acute or chronic Cholangitis
        Tumours: benign, malignant

CONGENITAL ANOMALIES

Pathology

The commonest finding is a bi-locular appearance of the gall-bladder (Phrygian cap) caused by a congenital fold or partial septum. Double or bi-lobed gall-bladders and true diverticula also occur. Agenesis is rare but malposition is not infrequent. Atresia of the bile ducts may also occur.

Clinical features

Although these anomalies are both common and complex they rarely, if ever, give rise to symptoms in adult life. However, they are important for the radiologist in interpreting films on cholecystography.

CHOLELITHIASIS

Aetiology

Biliary calculi may consist of pure pigment (bilirubin), pure

The Biliary Tract

cholesterol or a mixture of both. Calcium may or may not be deposited simultaneously. Apart from pure pigment stones which may be indicative of excessive haemolysis, distinction between the varieties of stone is usually not of clinical importance. The reasons for their development remain controversial, but since gallbladder bile is a supersaturated solution of bilirubin and cholesterol, it is perhaps surprising that crystallisation is not even more common.

Pathology

1 If the stones grow to a sufficient size before chance causes them to enter the cystic duct, they will be unable to pass easily and will then give rise to colic.
2 When they impact in the common duct they may cause obstructive jaundice.
3 Other symptoms result from biliary tract infection which itself may have been the initial cause of the calculus formation.

Clinical features

1 The classical symptom is right-sided subcostal pain of a colicky nature, which radiates through to the subscapular area on the same side.
2 Pain is usually intermittent or episodic.
3 There may be a background of dyspepsia after meals but when present, this suggests that there is also biliary infection.
 Although the formation of stones in the biliary tract is very common in many cases these give rise to no symptoms.

Investigations

1 Plain X-ray of the gallbladder area will demonstrate radio-opaque stones.
2 Oral cholecystography will demonstrate the majority of stones which appear as filling defects in the gallbladder. Radiolucent stones in a normally functioning gallbladder can be more easily demonstrated by taking one film in the standing position. The calculi then range themselves

in a line across the gallbladder and become more readily visible.
3 Intravenous cholangiography is preferable for demonstrating calculi within the common duct but as this technique does not demonstrate the gallbladder so well it must be considered complementary to oral cholecystography.

Differential diagnosis

Many other conditions may simulate biliary colic, especially hiatus hernia, peptic ulcer and myocardial ischaemia and it is important to consider these other possibilities before ascribing the symptoms to the incidental finding of gall stones on X-ray.

Treatment

It must be reiterated that the majority of these calculi are entirely asymptomatic and so their discovery does not necessarily indicate an operative approach but since there is no known drug capable of dissolving gall stones *in situ* and because symptoms once they have occurred are likely to recur, the advantages of prophylactic surgery must be evaluated in each case.

INFECTION

Acute cholecystitis

Aetiology

This condition is not common and probably accounts for no more than 1—5% of all biliary tract disease.
The usual precipitating factor is obstruction and a stone impacted in the ampulla is a frequent finding.

Other rare causes are:
1 Torsion of the duct
2 Involvement of the duct in a peri-duodenitis
3 Infiltration of the area by neoplasm.

Clinical features

Symptoms are sudden and usually unheralded and consist of

The Biliary Tract

severe right subcostal pain radiating through to the subscapular region. Nausea and vomiting are prominent features, together with fever and tachycardia. An acutely sensitive and distended gallbadder may be palpated and occasionally there is shoulder tip pain referred from diaphragmatic irritation.

Investigations

1 A high polymorphonuclear leucocytosis is usual
2 Radiology is only sometimes helpful, stones being seen in a plain X-ray in about 10% of cases.

Treatment

As with the appendix, the gallbladder possesses a vulnerable blood supply and so gangrene and perforation may occur.

1 In severe cases surgical relief is an urgent necessity and laparotomy should be performed without delay.
2 Many cases are less dramatically severe and some have already had symptoms for several days before seeking aid. In these a conservative approach is justified and cholecystectomy should be delayed until the patient's general and local condition permits a more adequate exploration of the field and in particular of the common duct.

In these patients treatment consists of:
   (a) Nursing in an upright position
   (b) Maintenance of continuous gastric aspiration with the aim of minimising gallbladder activity
   (c) Maintenance of water and electrolyte balance with intravenous fluids.
   (d) Antibotic therapy with Ampicillin or Tetracycline as both these are concentrated in bile.
   (e) Strong analgesics, such as Pethidine 100 mgms. or Papaverine 30 mgms.—60 mgms., may be necessary. It must be borne in mind that opiates tend to increase spasm of the sphincter of Oddi and further impair biliary drainage.

Chronic cholecystitis

Aetiology

This is more common than acute cholecystitis and is frequently, although not invariably, associated with stones.

Pathology

The wall of the gallbladder may be either mildly infiltrated with inflammatory cells or almost entirely replaced by fibrous tissue. Function is usually, but by no means always, impaired and it is a common error to dismiss the presence of infection on the evidence of apparently satisfactory cholecystography.

Clinical features

The history is usually prolonged with dyspepsia occurring after meals but not necessarily with fatty foods. Gallbladder dyspepsia is variable in degree and lacks the true periodicity that is characteristic of peptic ulceration. Discomfort is most often in the right subcostal area and may radiate through to the subscapular region on the same side. Occasionally the pain is felt centrally in the epigastrium, but even in these instances the area of tenderness is usually still to the right of the mid-line.

It is rare for a mass to be felt because the gallbladder is small due to chronic fibrosis.

Jaundice, if present, is almost always an indication that stones are present and that they have escaped to become lodged in the common bile duct.

Investigations

1. A moderate polymorphonuclear leucocytosis is usual but not invariable.
2. Hepatic function tests are not disturbed except in the rare instances of common duct occlusion, in which case there is an obstructive pattern.
3. Cholecystography is a valuable aid to diagnosis and provided adequate contrast medium is absorbed, failure to see the gallbladder suggests disease. Normal concentration of the dye however does not entirely exclude disease.

Treatment

1. Patients who have chronic cholecystitis associated with stones should be offered cholecystectomy after the phase of acute inflammation has been controlled.
2. Patients who are not suitable for surgery or who do not

have stones may respond surprisingly well to a medical régime, the aim of which is to re-establish function at the same time as eradicating infection.

The patient is first warned that initially the treatment may result in temporary accentuation of symptoms. He is then instructed to broaden his diet gradually, to take small quantities at frequent intervals and to include some form of fat in each meal with the object of stimulating the gallbladder. Antibiotics are simultaneously administered (Tetracycline 250 mgms. q.d.s.) and the dosage maintained for longer than usual (14—21 days at least). Bile flow from the liver can also be encouraged by the administration of bile salts (Dehydrocholine 1 q.d.s.) and later gallbladder activity can be still further stimulated with small repeated doses of Mag. Sulph (drm. 1 t.d.s.).

This régime however is strongly contraindicated in the presence of acute biliary infection since stimulation of the gallbladder in these cases will predispose to perforation.

Cholangitis

Aetiology

Cholangitis may follow:
1. Cholecystitis especially if partial obstruction of the common duct has occurred as a result of trauma or fibrosis.
2. Stones or tumours situated at the ampulla of Vater.
3. Passage of intestinal parasites from the duodenum up the duct.
4. Obstruction of the common duct by disease in the head of the pancreas.

Pathology

The infection ascends via the biliary channels to reach the liver and the organisms may gain direct access to the circulation, producing septicaemia.

Primary cholangitis is considerably less common and some authorities challenge its existence as a separate entity. Others postulate a haematogenous source for the infection and suggest that viruses, as well as bacteria, may sometimes be responsible.

If the infection is uncontrolled, intrahepatic abscesses may develop and if the chronic obstructive element predominates, a biliary type of cirrhosis can develop.

Clinical features

1 The patient presents with recurrent episodes of jaundice often accompanied by severe rigors and distressing pruritus.
2 Pain can be severe but in some cases there may be surprisingly little discomfort and the liver need not be tender to palpation.
3 Nausea and vomiting are frequent.
4 Weight loss may be profound.

Treatment

Antibiotic therapy should be both intensive and prolonged and as with all biliary and hepatic infections, broad spectrum antibiotics that are concentrated by the liver and in the bile are most effective.

Surgery should be undertaken since it is essential to relieve obstruction and to establish free biliary drainage.

TUMOURS

Benign lesions

These are of little clinical importance but they occasionally give rise to difficulties in differential diagnosis, since they simulate either calculi or malignancy.

Small intra-vesical polyps are fairly common and they may be either papillomatous, adenomatous or consist principally of cholesterol.

Carcinoma

Aetiology

Primary gallbladder malignancy ranks sixth in frequency among carcinoma of the alimentary tract. The sex incidence is comparable with that of cholelithiasis, being four to one in favour of the female. Its maximum age incidence is in the sixth decade and 95% are associated with gall stones.

Pathology

Both adenomatous and squamous types occur but the former constitute the majority (80—90%).

Clinical features

1 Clinically carcinoma is rarely recognised until well advanced as it is relatively asymptomatic in the early stages.
2 There may be a preceding history of cholecystitis.

Carcinoma of the Ampulla of Vater

This deserves separate mention for although clinically it closely simulates carcinoma of the head of the pancreas, it can sometimes be diagnosed sufficiently early for radical surgery to be successful.

Jaundice is an early sign and at the same time there is intestinal blood loss. Usually this can only be detected chemically but occasionally the biliary obstruction and bleeding are severe enough to give a 'silver stool'. This is a combination of acholia and melaena, i.e. the clay colour of biliary obstruction and the black of altered blood.

In general the picture is that of common duct obstruction in the absence of cholecystitis, with a distended gallbladder giving rise to a palpable mass in the right upper quadrant.

CHAPTER 8

THE PANCREAS

Classification of pancreatic disorders:
1 **Congenital**
    (a) **Developmental anomalies.**
        (i) **Duct variations**
        (ii) **Annular pancreas**
        (iii) **Pancreatic heterotopia**
    (b) **Inherited disease**
        Cystic fibrosis
2 **Trauma**
3 **Inflammation**
    (a) **Acute (necrotising or haemorrhagic) pancreatitis**
    (b) **Subacute relapsing pancreatitis**
    (c) **Chronic pancreatitis**
    (d) **Pancreatic lithiasis**
4 **Tumours**
    (a) **Islet cell adenomata**
        (i) **insulin secreting**
        (ii) **non-insulin secreting**
    (b) **Malignant—adenocarcinoma.**

CONGENITAL

(a) **Developmental anomalies**
(i) Duct variations.
    Variations in the anatomy of the pancreatic ductal system are very common and the relationship of the main pancreatic duct to the common bile duct at the Ampulla of Vater is important. Often these two ducts share a common channel for the final few

millimetres of their course and when this happens bile may regurgitate into the substance of the pancreas.

Apart from this, ductal anomalies are of little importance.

(ii) Annular pancreas.

Annular pancreas is the term used to describe the situation when the head of the pancreas partially or completely surrounds the second or descending part of the duodenum. Although autopsy evidence reveals that this is by no means an uncommon state of affairs, it only rarely gives any clinical evidence of its existence.

Clinical features

When symptoms do occur they are:
1 Vomiting due to high intestinal obstruction
2 Jaundice may occur if the common bile duct becomes involved.

Treatment

Operation is clearly necessary and a by-pass procedure is preferred to a simple division of the encircling ring. The latter procedure carries a risk of producing a pancreatic fistula.

(iii) Pancreatic Heterotopia (accessory pancreatic rests)

In the great majority of cases these isolated fragments of pancreatic tissue are located in the submucosa of the stomach or duodenum in close proximity to the pylorus.

It is a rare condition but the symptoms closely mimic those of peptic ulcer. The condition is described at greater length in Chapter 18.

(b) Inherited disease

Cystic fibrosis (mucoviscidosis)

This genetically determined condition consists of disturbed activity in the goblet or mucus producing cells.

As well as in the pancreas, mucus secretion throughout the whole length of the intestinal canal, in the lungs, and salivary glands may be affected. The secretion from the sweat glands of the skin is also altered and contains an excess of sodium and chloride.

The ducts of the mucous glands become obstructed with the abnormally viscid mucus with the result that not only is there impaired secretion but also cystic change in the ducts and secondary infection.

The condition most frequently presents in childhood but some less severe cases succeed in reaching adult life before being detected.

Clinical features

The two major features are:
1. Pancreatic insufficiency (weight loss and steatorrhoea).
2. Recurrent respiratory infection (bronchiolitis, pneumonia, bronchiectasis).

Other features are:
1. Meconium ileus may be the presenting picture in the neonatal period.
2. Prolapse of the rectum or swelling of the sub-maxillary glands may occur occasionally in infants.
3. Circulatory prostration can occur due to profound sodium and chloride depletion via the abnormal sweat glands. This is more likely to be encountered in the summer months.

Investigations

1. Examination of the sweat.
   The sweat will contain a high sodium and chloride content (above 60—80 meq./litre for either sodium or chloride). Agar plates impregnated with silver nitrate are a useful screening test in adults.
2. Faecal fat estimations may demonstrate steatorrhoea.
3. Pancreatic function tests are difficult in children but can show qualitative differences in secretion.
4. Chest X-rays may show secondary lung changes of bronchiectasis.

Treatment

1. As far as intestinal symptoms are concerned this consists of replacement therapy. Large doses of pancreatic extract may have to be given and sometimes insulin is also necessary.
2. The lung changes lead to bronchiectasis and recurrent infections for which repeated courses or long term administration of antibiotics are needed.

With care and perseverance many of the children suffering from this disease can be brought safely to adult life without any overt evidence of maldevelopment.

TRAUMA

In spite of the relative inaccessibility of the pancreas, injuries can occur. Contusion accounts for the majority of cases, produced usually by the steering wheel in car accidents.

Clinical features

Symptoms of contusion damage need not be immediate and they are frequently overshadowed by the other incidental injuries. Necrotic pancreatitis may develop insidiously.

In all cases of direct abdominal injury the possibilty of a pseudocyst developing subsequently should be anticipated and a careful follow-up maintained.

Treatment

In the acute stage conservative management is preferred but laparotomy may be required to exclude other intra-abdominal injury.

INFLAMMATION

Acute (necrotising or haemorrhagic) pancreatitis

In acute pancreatitis tissue necrosis occurs due to escape of activated proteolytic enzymes. Oedema is always marked and haemorrhage into the gland may be severe.

Aetiology

The predisposing causes of pancreatitis are impairment of secretory drainage and stimulus to excessive exocrine secretion and there are many possible aetiological factors but the two of outstanding importance are:
1 Bilary tract infection.
   Pre-existing chronic cholecystitis accounts for the majority of cases occurring in this country, as it predisposes to

regurgitation of infected bile into the pancreatic duct. This is more likely to occur when the terminal duct is shared by both biliary and pancreatic systems.

2 Alcohol.

Relationship between alcohol and acute pancreatitis is undeniable but there need not be an excessive intake. In some individuals a consistent correlation between the ingestion of even a small quantity of alcohol and a subsequent rise in the serum amylase level can be demonstrated. There may be other minor additional factors such as transient duodenal oedema concerned in the production of an acute attack.

Other less common aetiological associations are:

1 Pancreatic duct obstruction due to calculus, tumour, worm infestation etc.
2 Post-operative (abdominal surgery)
3 Hyperparathyroidism
4 Steroid administration
5 Hereditary acute pancreatitis
6 Primary bacterial or virus infection (mumps produces acute oedematous pancreatitis)
7 Allergic reaction.

Clinical features

1 Exceedingly severe pain is the outstanding symptom. The onset is sudden and although it may follow a large meal, more often than not it is entirely unheralded. It is central epigastric in site and radiates through to the mid-back with an unusually penetrating quality.
2 It is often accompanied by shock, so that although the patient is febrile, the pulse is thready and the blood pressure low.
3 The abdomen is tender and sometimes considerable distension occurs. True board-like rigidity is uncommon.
4 Nausea and vomiting can occur and the overall picture closely simulates that of a perforated ulcer from which it can often only be distinguished at emergency laparotomy.
5 Blue discolouration may be seen in the loin and around the umbilicus (due to retro- and intra-peritoneal haemorrhage)

but this only develops after some days and is therefore of little value in the early differential diagnosis.

Investigations

1 An elevated serum amylase level (over 500 Somogyi units) in a specimen of blood taken before the administration of analgesics (especially morphia) is highly suggestive. Raised serum amylase levels may result from peptic ulcer on the pancreas or from a dose of morphine. Serum lipase levels rise later.
2 Leucocytosis is moderate.
3 Transient hyperglycaemia occurs in a small percentage of cases.
4 Hypocalcaemia is usually of ominous significance and is due to calcium deposition in fat necrosis.
5 Changes can occur in the electrocardiograph and these do not necessarily indicate a coronary lesion, although this may occur as a complication.

Treatment

1 Continuous gastric aspiration should be instituted immediately. The objective is to prevent acid entering the duodenum and stimulating pancreatic secretory activity via the secretin mechanism.
2 The administration of full doses of Atropine or another anticholinergic agent such as Probanthine will further inhibit enzyme production. This may also help to relieve the situation by reducing spasm in the Sphincter of Oddi.
3 Shock is countered by means of intravenous therapy using plasma until suitable blood can be obtained and crossmatched.
4 Pain is controlled by Pethidine 100 mgms. or Papaverine 60 mgms. These agents are less likely than morphine to produce sphincter spasm and an increase of intraductal pressure. Adequate control of the very severe pain is often difficult to achieve and if facilities are available, continuous epidural block may be more successful.
5 Specific antisecretory agents have been advocated such as Acetazolamide (Diamox) 250—500 mgm. twice daily for suppression of both secretion volume and the bicarbonate

output. Trasylol is claimed, but not proved to be an even more effective trypsin inhibitor. It is administered intravenously in large doses (100,000 units daily). Careful watch should be maintained for possible anaphylactic reactions.
6 Insulin may be required to compensate a temporary diabetic state and intravenous calcium gluconate to counteract tetany.
7 Hydrocortisone is indicated in all severe cases, if only to forestall adrenal exhaustion.
8 It is probably wise to prescribe a broad spectrum antibiotic, even in the absence of any frank infection.

After recovery it is most important to institute thorough investigations, particularly of the biliary tract. In addition to cholecystography and cholangiography, it may be informative to take serum amylase levels before and after standard doses of morphia and alcohol and possible even after certain foodstuffs which the patients themselves have found to be provocative.

Subacute relapsing pancreatitis—chronic pancreatitis—pancreatic lithiasis

These three conditions are best considered together since the background is common to all, with biliary tract disease, and alcohol intake as the most frequent factors involved. The intensity, the frequency and the periodicity of symptoms however differ.

Pathology

Once established pancreatitis tends to run a progressive course in spite of the removal of aetiological factors. There is progressive destruction and loss of both exocrine and endocrine secretions with replacement fibrosis and calcification.

Clinical features

1 Pain. The clinical picture is extremely variable and may consist of anything from transient episodes of post-prandial discomfort to repeated full scale attacks of acute pancreatitis.

Less often the symptoms are continuous with persistent and intractable central epigastric and mid-back pain. Such

The Pancreas

patients run a grave risk of becoming addicted to drugs since only opiates give adequate relief.
2. Diabetes may develop due to islet cell destruction.
3. Weight loss and general debility may result from steatorrhoea due to lack of pancreatic lipase.
4. Jaundice may result from fibrotic obstruction of the common bile duct.
5. Malignancy may develop insidiously.

Investigations
1. Plain X-ray of the abdomen may show pancreatic calcification or stones in the biliary tract.
2. Pancreatic function tests employing secretin and pancreozymin may be helpful in experienced hands.

Treatment
1. Low fat diet to reduce pancreatic stimulation and reduce steatorrhoea.
2. Replacement of pancreatic enzymes by frequent regular oral dosage.
3. Insulin therapy in cases of diabetes.
4. Relief of pain
   (i) in acute episodes with analgesics
   (ii) in intractable cases the extreme measure of total pancreatectomy may have to be considered, in spite of the initial risks and subsequent difficulties in management.
5. Removal of precipitating causes i.e. alcohol and gall stones.

TUMOURS

Islet-cell tumours

Classification

(a) Insulin secreting
(b) Non-insulin secreting.

(a) Insulin secreting adenomas
These are usually single, circumscribed and benign but they also can be multiple or diffuse and occasionally they are highly malignant.

Clinical features

Insulinomas can be responsible for periodic episodes of unusual and often violent behaviour as well as symptoms of hunger, faintness and sweating. The attacks frequently culminate in loss of consciousness.

Both physical and psychological features result from periods of profound hypoglycaemia and the patients themselves have usually discovered the protective value of eating sugar.

Investigations

Early recognition is important since any prolonged period of severe hypoglycaemia exposes the central nervous system to grave risk of permanent damage.

Confirmation of the diagnosis can usually be obtained by starving the patient for 12—24 hours but a longer test may be necessary. Failure of the serum glucose level to fall below 50 mg.% after 60 hours virtually excludes the diagnosis.

The administration of Tolbutamide intravenously intensifies the response giving an earlier result, but it is not without considerable risk and for this reason a syringe ready loaded with a 50% solution of glucose should be immediately available.

Treatment

This consists of surgical exploration and removal of the tumour. Occasionally the process is diffuse when a subtotal pancreatectomy may have to suffice, although the results of this procedure are satisfactory in only half the cases.

(b) Non-insulin secreting adenomas (Zollinger-Ellison syndrome)
   These tumours are rare but they are of particular interest because they produce gastrin which provokes excessive gastric secretion and this in turn results in peptic ulceration in atypical sites.

This condition is discussed at greater length in Chapter 18.

Malignant tumours of the pancreas

Whereas a few cases of malignancy develop as a sequel to recurrent or chronic pancreatitis, the majority arise *de novo*. These are chiefly adenocarcinomas but malignant change in islet cell tumours of both alpha and beta cell types are occasionally encountered.

Adenocarcinoma

Clinical features

The clinical picture varies according to the position of the growth in the pancreas. When situated in the head, pressure on the common bile duct may give rise to jaundice. A tumour in the body or tail may reach an advanced stage before giving any sign of its presence.

1. When jaundice does develop it is usually progressive and may be associated with the presence of a distended gallbladder.
2. Pain is indistinguishable from that of chronic pancreatitis and is dull and persistent.
3. Loss of weight is due to anorexia as a result of pain and rarely due to steatorrhoea.
4. Diabetes may develop in the elderly and be the first sign of carcinoma.
5. Superficial thrombophlebitis seems particularly likely to occur with pancreatic cancer.
6. Pancreatic malignancy is very frequently associated with psychological symptoms. These may sometimes amount to a personality change and such patients are often disproportionately miserable. For this reason, together with the lack of any positive diagnostic physical signs, they may be dismissed as neurotics.

Investigations

1. Barium meal may show widening and fixing of the duodenal loop, but this is a late sign and only occurs in those cases involving the head of the pancreas.
2. Serum amylase or lipase levels are rarely helpful since a large growth can be present without obstructing enzymatic outflow.
3. For the same reason duodenal intubation and analysis of exocrine secretion is equally disappointing as a diagnostic procedure.
4. Radioisotope scanning and selective angiography may be helpful but cannot detect small tumours easily.

Treatment

Although laparotomy may be undertaken early after symptoms develop, the lesion is all too frequently inoperable.

Partial or total pancreatectomy has a high mortality and morbidity and is usually precluded by the early local spread. Cholecysto-jejunostomy may be useful as a palliative measure to relieve jaundice and pruritis.

CHAPTER 9

THE SMALL INTESTINE

Classification of Disorders
1 **Infections**
    (a) **Bacterial**
    (b) **Protozoal**
    (c) **Viral**
    (d) **Fungal.**
2 **Peptic ulcer**
    (a) **Duodenal**
    (b) **Jejunal in Zollinger-Ellison syndrome**
    (c) **Ulceration in Meckel's diverticulum.**
3 **Diverticula**
    (a) **Duodenal diverticula**
    (b) **Multiple diverticulosis**
    (c) **Meckel's diverticulum**
4 **Inflammatory disease**
    Regional enterocolitis (Crohn's disease).
5 **Mucosal enzyme disorders**
    (a) **Gluten induced enteropathy**
    (b) **Tropical sprue**
    (c) **Disaccharidase deficiencies**
6 **Tumours**
    (a) **Benign**
    (b) **Malignant.**
7 **Mesenteric vascular occlusion**
    (a) **Arterial**
    (b) **Venous.**
8 **Mechanical problems**
    Obstruction, etc.
9 **Rarities**
    (a) **Whipple's disease**

84 *Lecture Notes on Gastroenterology*

(b) **Peutz-Jeghers syndrome**
(c) **Progressive systemic sclerosis**
(d) **Pneumatosis cystoides intestinalis.**

A number of the disorders listed above interfere with normal absorption and may present clinically with the malabsorption syndrome. This syndrome and a classification of its causes is also discussed separately in Chapter 10.

1 INFECTIONS

In the normal healthy person the lumen of the small intestine is unsuitable for the growth of organisms and therefore the contents are nearly sterile.

This state of affairs exists because of the bacteriocidal activity of the digestive juices. Gastric acidity is the initial barrier but pancreatic secretions are probably almost equally effective since patients suffering from achlorhydria do not seem unduly liable to intestinal infections.

Another condition unfavourable to bacterial proliferation is the speed of passage of the contents through the small intestine. Nevertheless in spite of these protective factors, under certain circumstances organisms do succeed in gaining a foothold in the small intestine.

The clinical features result from inflammation of the bowel wall and invasion of the circulation by organisms and their toxic products.

The whole subject of infection is dealt with at greater length in Chapter 12.

2 PEPTIC ULCER

Although duodenal ulceration is strictly a small intestinal disorder, this and jejunal ulcers are best considered together with gastric ulcer under the separate heading of peptic ulcer in Chapter 4. Meckel's diverticulum is described in the next section.

3 DIVERTICULA

In contrast to the diverticula of the large bowel, it is probable that all small intestinal diverticula have a congenital basis. For convenience the subject is best considered under three headings:
- (a) Duodenal diverticula
- (b) Small intestinal diverticulosis
- (c) Meckel's diverticulum.

(a) Duodenal Diverticula

Pathology

The duodenum is the commonest site for the development of diverticula and they usually project from the inner or concave border. They are most often free, but occasionally they lie embedded in the head of the pancreas.

Clinical features

They are usually disclosed incidentally at a Barium meal examination carried out for dyspepsia but the generally accepted view is that duodenal diverticula are invariably symptom free. They may, however, occasionally be responsible for haemorrhage and there is little doubt that the few that lie buried in the pancreas can be the seat of an inflammatory reaction.

Treatment

1. It is possible that very large specimens may give rise to an atypical episodic type of discomfort and there are reports of relief following surgical removal.
2. If the diverticula are associated with stasis and malabsorption, antibiotic therapy is worth a trial.

(b) Small Intestinal Diverticulosis

Pathology

There is great variability in both number, size and structure of these diverticula. Some consist of mucosa, sub-mucosa and serous coat only, while others possess a full muscle complement.

Clinical features

It is estimated that about 60% of the cases of multiple small intestinal diverticulosis are asymptomatic, but quite clearly they are potentially liable to complications such as obstruction, infection or perforation.

A proportion of cases suffer considerable disability in the form of anorexia, weight loss, increased intestinal activity and diarrhoea. A full malabsorption syndrome is more likely to result if the diverticula are situated in the jejunum. The cause is attributed to invasion of the lumen of the small intestine by bacteria which then compete for available supplies of essential metabolites.

Treatment

The condition is almost always far too extensive for total surgical clearance to be practicable but fortunately most cases can be maintained in a satisfactory state of health by means of a conservative régime. This consists of a low residue, high calorie diet, supplemented with vitamins and minerals. Folic acid should always be accompanied by Hydroxycobalamine (B_{12}) to prevent the development of sub-acute combined degeneration. Intermittent courses of antibiotics can prove beneficial in refractory cases.

(c) Meckel's Diverticulum

Aetiology

Incomplete regression of the vitelline (omphalo-mesenteric) duct results in a blind ended pouch of varying length, opening from the anti-mesenteric border of the ileum. This may or may not remain connected to the umbilicus by means of a fibrous cord.

Pathology

Meckel's diverticula are lined with functioning gastric type mucosa and so are potential sites for the development of peptic ulceration.

Clinical features

The presence of a Meckel's diverticulum is fairly common

The Small Intestine

(1%—3%) but the great majority are entirely silent throughout life. If and when peptic ulceration does develop, the clinical picture may closely resemble the more common duodenal lesion with the classical periodic dyspepsia. However, the pain tends to be peri-umbilical rather than epigastric, although it may still have a relationship to food. Complications can occur and may present as:

1. Symptomless melaena.
2. A general peritonitis due to perforation.
3. Obstruction due to a loop of bowel becoming caught up by the fibrous band which sometimes connects the diverticulum to the umbilicus.

Treatment

This is only necessary when complications develop and consists of surgical removal of the diverticulum.

4 INFLAMMATORY DISEASE

Regional Entero-colitis

Although this entity was first described by Crohn as a small intestinal disease (terminal ileitis), it is now widely recognised that it may involve any part of the intestinal canal from the stomach to the rectum. It is a non-specific granulomatous inflammatory process of as yet undiscovered aetiology and is fully discussed in Chapter 15.

5 MUCOSAL ENZYME DISORDERS

(a) Gluten induced enteropathy (Coeliac disease, idiopathic steatorrhoea)

Aetiology

This disorder is due to a reaction of the small intestinal mucosa to peptides contained in gliadin. Gliadin is found in the protein of wheat (gluten) and to a lesser extent in rye, oats and barley. Due to the unusual properties of wheat protein, the structure of the responsible peptide has not yet been fully resolved. It is not yet known whether the mucosal changes are due to sensitivity to the peptide or to toxic damage caused by the peptide in the absence of the appropriate catabolic enzyme.

Pathology

The mucosa of the small intestine looks abnormal both macroscopically and microscopically. In severe cases the whole small bowel may be affected, the changes decreasing in severity from duodenum to ileum. In less severe cases or those under treatment, only the proximal bowel may be affected.

The mucosal changes are:

Macroscopically:
  (i) The surface is flat with absence of differentiation into villi.
  (ii) The mouths of the crypts are visible and the mucosal surface may be lobulated (mosaic pattern).

Microscopically:
  (i) The epithelial cells lose their normal tall columnar appearance and become cuboid or irregular.
  (ii) The microvilli are irregular and stunted.
  (iii) There is an increased infiltration of round cells and plasma cells in the lamina propria.
  (iv) The depth of crypts and number of glands are increased.

These appearances may become less marked after treatment but only rarely does the mucosa revert entirely to normal. The degree of the severity of the steatorrhoea and the clinical illness is likely to be greater the more the small bowel is affected but the correlation is not exact.

Clinical features

Patients may present:
1 In early childhood after weaning with stunted growth, protuberant belly, diarrhoea and irritability.
2 In adolescence with similar but less obvious symptoms and signs.
3 In adult life at any age and usually with symptoms of deficiency due to malabsorption associated with inter-

The Small Intestine

mittent or low grade diarrhoea. Folic acid deficiency and anaemia may be precipitated by pregnancy and severe osteoporosis may be found in the elderly.

The features of the malabsorption syndrome are described in detail in Chapter 10.

Investigations

1. A Barium meal and follow-through may show a malabsorption pattern with dilated segments of small bowel and a coarse mucosal appearance.
2. Peroral small bowel biopsy will show an abnormal mucosa.
3. Absorption studies particularly faecal fat estimation will confirm that malabsorption is occurring.
4. Blood studies will show evidence of anaemia and specific deficiencies.

Treatment

1. The first essential is to remove the deleterious effect of gluten by placing the patients on a gluten-free diet. For this careful explanation and expert dietetic advice is important.
2. Correlation of any anaemia and specific body deficiencies arising from the malabsorption should be carried out after the requirements have been assessed.
3. The symptoms of distension and diarrhoea may be improve by giving patients a low fat diet in the early stages.

(b) Tropical Sprue

Aetiology

This disorder occurs mainly in people living in certain tropical areas of the Far East and Central America. The aetiology is still not known but the following factors have been considered:

1. Altered bacterial flora with colonisation of the small gut.
2. Nutritional deficiency.
3. Specific harmful effect of local foodstuffs such as fats.

Pathology

The mucosa of the small intestine is abnormal:

1. The villi are shorter and blunter and the mucosa may have

a convoluted appearance. The mucosa is not as flat as in coeliac disease.
2 There is an increase in inflammatory cells including polymorphonuclear leucocytes in the submucosa.

Clinical features

These again are those of the malabsorption syndrome but symptoms due to folic acid deficiency with sore tongue, stomatitis and macrocytic anaemia are common.

Investigations
1 A Barium follow-through will show a malabsorption pattern.
2 Peroral biopsy will show an abnormal mucosa.
3 Absorption and blood studies will confirm the presence and degree of deficiencies.

Treatment
1 Most patients respond well to oral folic acid.
2 Broad spectrum antibiotics have been used with success in some cases and are usually given with folic acid.
3 Some patients recover spontaneously on leaving the area.
4 Other specific deficiencies must be corrected with oral supplements of mineral and vitamins.

(c) Disaccharidase Deficiencies

Aetiology

Certain people are unable to split disaccharides because of specific intra-mucosal enzyme deficiencies. The three principal deficiencies are those of sucrase, maltase and lactase. These can occur:
1 As a primary disorder with congenital deficiency in the intestinal mucosal wall.
2 As a secondary phenomenon when there is a general mucosal cell disturbance due to other disease e.g. gluten enteropathy.

Pathology

There is no morphological abnormality in the small intestinal mucosa but histochemical and assay techniques will demonstrate an absence or deficiency of disaccharidase in mucosal specimens.

Clinical features
1. Patients may present in childhood or less commonly as adults with
    (a) diarrhoea and steatorrhoea
    (b) abdominal distension and flatulence
    (c) abdominal colic.
2. A number of people with enzyme deficiency will have no symptoms under normal circumstances but may develop them if presented with an excessive sugar load.

Investigations
1. A Barium follow-through is often normal although it may show a malabsorptive pattern. This may become more obvious by giving the specific sugar under investigation e.g. lactose together with the Barium.
2. Biochemical enzyme assays can be carried out on mucosal specimens obtained by peroral biopsy.
3. Specific sugar tolerance tests will be abnormal. False positive results however can be obtained in other mucosal disorders associated with malabsorption e.g. gluten enteropathy. Clinical symptoms are likely to be aggravated by performing these tests.

Treatment

This consists of placing the patient on a diet which does not contain the specific disaccharide. Adequate carbohydrate can be given in other forms.

6 TUMOURS

(a) Benign

Benign tumours of the small gut are exceedingly rare, they are usually solitary and they can be of different cell types e.g. lipoma, fibroma etc. Tumours can be multiple as in the Peutz-Jeghers syndrome of multiple adenomatosis associated with melanin pigmentation of the mucous membrane. This is described at greater length in Chapter 18.

(b) Malignant

Aetiology.

Although rare, when malignancy does occur, sarcomas or lymphomas are almost as common as carcinomas and for practical purposes malignant change can be considered not to occur in duodenal ulcers.

Secondary deposits from tumours outside the intestine e.g. melanoma, are met with on rare occasions.

The relationship between malignant disease and a flat jejunal mucosa (villous atrophy) is not yet defined but

1. Both lymphoma and carcinoma of the small bowel have occurred in patients with long-standing gluten enteropathy.
2. Local mucosal changes can occur in association with malignant tumours of the small intestine.
3. A flat mucosa has been found in association with malignant disease elsewhere in the body.
4. There is a higher incidence of carcinoma occurring in the gut or other sites such as the tonsil in patients with gluten enteropathy than in the normal population.

Clinical feaures

Tumours may present:

1. As incidental findings on X-ray.
2. With anaemia or frank haemorrhage.
3. With symptoms of obstruction.

Investigations

Barium follow-through may show filling defects indicating the presence of tumours.

Treatment

This consists of surgical removal of primary tumours where practicable.

The Small Intestine

7 MESENTERIC VASCULAR OCCLUSION

There is no invariable distinction between the clinical pictures produced by obstruction of the mesenteric arterial or venous systems, differences in symptoms being more closely related to the degree of vascular involvement. Intravascular thrombosis is the usual cause but occasionally occlusion may result from arterial embolism.

The superior mesenteric vessels are more frequently involved than the inferior so that the small intestine is more likely to be affected than the caecum or ascending colon.

Clinical features

1. In minor instances there may be no more than intermittent abdominal discomfort following food (abdominal angina or mid-gut ischaemia). This however usually indicates atherosclerotic narrowing of the mesenteric vessels rather than occlusion.
2. In more extensive disease abdominal pain is accompanied by distension and bloodstained diarrhoea. There may also be superficial abdominal tenderness due to peritoneal involvement.
3. Massive infarction produces a very dramatic picture which can closely simulate acute pancreatitis. The pain is exceedingly severe and is accompanied by shock. Vomiting, bloodstained diarrhoea and perforation may occur.

Investigations

Selective angiography may be helpful in subacute or chronic cases.

Treatment

(a) In infarction.

Urgent surgery is required and mortality is high. Malabsorption may occur later if extensive resection is unavoidable.

(b) In chronic ischaemia.
Where a definite diagnosis is made, surgical removal of the obstruction may be possible in some cases. Unfortunately most patients are elderly and have other serious manifestations of vascular disease e.g. coronary ischaemia.

8 SMALL INTESTINAL OBSTRUCTION

The following are the most common causes of obstruction:
Adhesions and bands
Intussusception and volvulus
Hernia—simple or strangulated
Chronic inflammation—Crohn's disease or tuberculosis
Tumours—benign or malignant
Paralytic ileus
Mesenteric vascular occlusion.

Clinical features

Griping abdominal pain, distension and constipation are the cardinal features with vomiting as an early manifestation.

The onset is usually sudden and unheralded. Later the pain becomes constant especially if strangulation of the blood supply has occurred. In this case there is inevitable peritoneal involvement and signs of toxaemia develop.

Investigations

A straight X-ray of the abdomen is of great assistance as it reveals the distended coils of gut with multiple fluid levels.

Treatment

This consists of surgical relief of the obstruction. There is often disturbed water and electrolyte balance which requires urgent correction as far as possible pre-operatively by intravenous fluids.

9 RARETIES

(a) **Whipple's disease**
(b) **Peutz-Jeghers syndrome**
(c) **Progressive systemic sclerosis**
(d) **Pneumatosis cystoides intestinalis.**

These are discussed in Chapter 18.

CHAPTER 10
THE 'MALABSORPTION' SYNDROME

Aetiology

The fundamental basis of the syndrome is faulty assimilation of proteins, carbohydrates, fats, minerals and vitamins by the small intestine and it may result from a variety of causes, the more important of which are conveniently grouped as follows:

Classification:
1 **Alterations in small intestinal anatomy**
    (a) Resection
    (b) Short circuiting
    (c) Blind loops
    (d) Multiple diverticula
    (e) Post-gastrectomy.
2 **Disturbances of intraluminal digestion**
    (a) Deficiency of pancreatic enzymes
    (b) Bacterial colonisation of the small gut
    (c) Massive gastric hypersecretion (Zollinger-Ellison syndrome).
3 **Defects of mucosal cell function**
    (a) Gluten enteropathy (coeliac disease)
    (b) Tropical sprue
    (c) Disaccharidase deficiencies
    (d) Drug toxicity i.e. neomycin or phenindione.
4 **Physical changes in the gut wall**
    (a) Inflammatory:
        (i) tuberculous enteritis
        (ii) regional enteritis
    (b) Proliferative:
        (i) leukaemias
        (ii) reticuloses (lymphomas etc.)

The 'Malabsorption' Syndrome

    (c) **Infiltrative:**
       (i) **amyloidosis**
       (ii) **Whipple's disease**
       (iii) **progressive systemic sclerosis.**
5 **Changes in neurological supply**
    (a) **Vagotomy**
    (b) **Diabetes Mellitus.**
6 **Changes in vascular and lymph supply**
    (a) **Arterial ischaemia**
    (b) **Chronic venous congestion**
    (c) **Congenital lymphangiectasia.**

Clinical features

Whatever the underlying cause of the absorptive insufficiency, the clinical picture is frequently similar.

In cases of recent onset abdominal and bowel symptoms may be predominant but long standing cases may present a complex picture due to multiple deficiencies.

1 Weight loss is usual and may be severe and in children growth will be stunted.
2 The stools are characteristically pale, bulky, offensive, float on the surface and are difficult to flush away. In less severe cases however the stools may appear normal.

    Diarrhoea does not always occur.
3 The abdomen is protuberant in children but distension is less marked in adults.
4 Abdominal discomfort and borborygmi are common but pain is not a feature unless associated with the primary condition.
5 Symptoms and signs of specific deficiencies are commonly seen:

    fatigue due to anaemia or hypokalaemia
    oedema due to hypoprotainaemia or anaemia
    tetany due to hypocalcaemia
    haemorrhages due to hypoprothrombinaemia
    koilonychia due to iron deficiency
    glossitis and stomatitis due to folic acid deficiency
    bone pain due to hypocalcaemia
    increased liability to infections due to globulin deficiency.
6 Endocrine activity may be depressed and present as inhibi-

tion of growth, hypothermia and hypotension. Pigmentation of the skin and mucous membranes may result from hypoadrenalism.
7 Mental changes occur particularly in gluten enteropathy. The irritability and difficulty in management of these patients is often strikingly improved after treatment.

Investigations

These are performed
- (a) To confirm that malabsorption is occurring.
- (b) To assess the degree of deficiency resulting from the malabsorption.
- (c) To diagnose the primary cause of malabsorption.

These aims are clearly not entirely dissociated from each other since for instance low serum levels of iron indicate deficiency but also, in the absence of obvious blood loss, suggest malabsorption.

In the same way a follow-through X-ray may show a malabsorption pattern (see below) and also demonstrate the primary cause e.g. jejunal diverticulosis.

(a) The most widely used indices of malabsorption are:
1 Faecal fat estimation.
   The normal average daily fat excretion on a diet containing at least 75 gms. fat is less than 5 gms. measured over a three or five day period. Figures above this level indicate further investigations are necessary.
2 Xylose absorption test.
   Less than 20% excretion of a 25 gm. oral dose within five hours suggests a mucosal defect.

Specific absorption tests for other elements can be and often are done but are not used routinely for the diagnosis of general malabsorption.

(b) Assessment of deficiency.
1 Blood Picture.
   There is usually a moderate or severe anaemia which may be frankly macrocytic or of mixed type due to combined deficiencies of iron, folic acid and vitamin B_{12}. The blood levels of these three substances can be measured and will indicate the degree of deficiency.

2 Serum Chemistry.
Estimation of the levels of serum proteins, electrolytes and calcium will give further indication of the systemic effects of the malabsorption.

(c) Diagnosis of the primary lesion.
This may be obvious from the history or from examination but X-rays and gut biopsy will usually be required at least for the confirmation if not the making of the diagnosis.

1 Radiography.
A Barium meal and follow-through is essential and may both demonstrate the primary cause of the malabsorption as well as showing a 'malabsorption pattern'. This comprises dilatation and alteration of calibre of segments of small bowel, a coarse mucosal pattern and flocculation of the Barium. It should be noted that the presence of flocculation depends greatly on the type of Barium used in the examination and care must be taken in interpreting this sign.

A plain X-ray of the skeleton may show radiological osteoporosis which in these cases is due to deficiency of both calcium and protein.

2 Small bowel biopsy.
Biopsies can be taken at laparotomy or through peroral suction biopsy instruments. Several types are available and with some several specimens can be obtained at one intubation. The biopsy material can be examined histologically or chemically for evidence of structural and enzymatic disorders. These techniques are of particular value in diffuse mucosal disorders such as gluten enteropathy, disaccharidase deficiency and lymphangiectasia. It is often of considerable help to have a normal biopsy thus excluding such diseases.

Differential Diagnosis

In children fibrocystic disease of the pancreas (mucoviscidosis) should be suspected if there is an associated liability to chest infections and a high sodium chloride content in sweat; congenital lymphangiectasia of the gut may be associated with lymphangiectasia elsewhere e.g. face or limbs; coeliac disease can be confirmed by gut biopsy and the response to gluten withdrawal from the diet.

In adults pancreatic enzyme insufficiency may be difficult to prove but an associated diabetic glucose tolerance curve is highly suggestive of pancreatic disease.

The surgical and anatomical causes of malabsorption are usually diagnosed from the previous history and can be confirmed with Barium studies. These will also demonstrate diverticulosis and most cases of regional enteritis which are sufficiently extensive to interfere with absorption.

Disaccharidase deficiences can be proven by the appropriate (lactose, maltose, sucrose) absorption tests and enzyme studies of gut mucosa obtained by biopsy.

In the reticuloses and occasionally in Whipple's disease, an enlarged lymph node may be available for biopsy.

The leukaemias are revealed by blood or bone marrow examination.

Systemic sclerosis is rarely present in the gut without also involving the skin (scleroderma).

Treatment

The principles of treatment are:
1 To treat or remove the primary cause as far as possible e.g.:
    pancreatic extract by mouth in pancreatic disease;
    a gluten-free diet in coeliac disease;
    antibiotic therapy in diverticulosis;
    correction of anatomical derangement.
2 Where specific treatment or removal of the primary lesion is not possible e.g. previous extensive resections, to try and overcome the malabsorption by increasing the intake of essential foodstuffs.
3 In all cases to replace the specific deficiencies demonstrated by examination and investigations. Both intravenous and intramuscular therapy is often necessary.
4 To reduce the symptoms associated with steatorrhoea and intestinal fermentation i.e. the distension, offensive stools and diarrhoea. In the early stages of treatment at least, most of the patients with steatorrhoea feel better with a reduced dietary fat intake. Where the primary cause is treatable, a normal diet may be introduced later.

CHAPTER 11

ANAEMIA AND THE ALIMENTARY TRACT

Anaemia caused by gastrointestinal disease may be due to:
   (a) **Loss of whole blood**
   (b) **Impaired assimilation of haemopoietic factors.**

(A) BLOOD LOSS

Classification of causes
1 **Abnormal blood vessels**
   (a) **Oesophageal varices**
   (b) **Haemorrhoids**
   (c) **Multiple hereditary telangiectasia.**
2 **Hiatus hernia**
3 **Peptic ulceration**
   (a) **Stomach or duodenum**
   (b) **Jejunum in Zollinger-Ellison syndrome**
   (c) **Meckel's diverticulum.**
4 **Diverticulosis**
   (a) **Duodenum**
   (b) **Colon.**
5 **Inflammatory disorders**
   (a) **Regional enterocolitis**
   (b) **Ulcerative colitis.**
6 **Infections**
   (a) **Typhoid**
   (b) **Tuberculosis**
   (c) **Amoebic dysentery**
   (d) **Bacillary dysentery.**

7 Infections
  (a) Ankylostomiasis
  (b) Bilharziasis.
8 Metabolic uraemia
9 Blood disorders
  (a) Leukaemias
  (b) Anticoagulant therapy.
10 Benign or malignant tumours of any part of the gastrointestinal tract
11 Iatrogenic
  (a) Aspirin
  (b) Instrumentation.

Pathology

The anaemia will be initially normocytic and normochromic but if loss continues body iron stores become depleted and a microcytic hypochromic anaemia results.

(B) IMPAIRED ASSIMILATION OF HAEMOPOIETIC FACTORS

Classification of causes.
1 Inadequate intake due to
  (a) General malnutrition
  (b) Individual deficiencies, iron, B_{12}, folic acid, etc.
2 Inadequate absorption due to
  (a) Previous surgery
    (i) gastrectomy
    (ii) small gut resection
    (iii) short circuits, etc.
  (b) Pancreatic and biliary disease
    (i) pancreatitis
    (ii) biliary duct obstruction.
  (c) Small intestinal mucosal defects
    (i) gluten-induced enteropathy
    (ii) regional enteritis, etc.
  (d) Intestinal stasis
    (i) diverticulosis
    (ii) blind loops, etc.

Anaemia and the Alimentary Tract

(e) Absence of the intrinsic factor
  (i) pernicious anaemia
  (ii) carcinoma stomach.
(f) Competition from parasites
  Infestations with Dibothriocephalus latus.

Pathology

All the haematinic agents may be involved in dietary deficiency but relative to requirements the body stores of iron and folic acid are less than those of Vitamin B_{12}.

1. Nutritional deficiency therefore commonly presents as a hypochromic anaemia due to the negative iron balance although there is frequently an underlying folic acid deficiency as well.
2. Partial gastrectomy, particularly of the Bilroth II and Ploya types, commonly results in an iron deficiency anaemia (although more than one factor may be involved) largely due to impaired absorption of food iron.
3. Total gastrectomy inevitably results in a macrocytic type of anaemia due to lack of intrinsic factor secretion which in turn leads to an inability to absorb dietary B_{12}. Anaemia does not develop immediately as normal hepatic stores are adequate for up to three years.
4. Apart from haemorrhage and iron deficiency states, anaemias of gastro-intestinal origin are predominantly megaloblastic and may arise as follows:
   (a) In addition to the common form of pernicious anaemia associated with gastric atrophy there is a genetically determined disorder, juvenile pernicious anaemia, due to absence of the intrinsic factor.
   (b) In small intestinal diverticula and blind loops there may be stagnation allowing bacteria to establish themselves and compete for the small available supplies of Vitamin B_{12}.
   (c) The fish tapeworm Dibothriocephalus latus consumes Vitamin B_{12} so that infestation with this parasite can produce a macrocytic anaemia.
   (d) In patients with mucosal abnormalities such as coeliac disease, idiopathic steatorrhoea and tropical sprue, there is poor absorption of folic acid and of Vitamin B_{12}.

Clinical features

1. Fatigue, exertional dyspnoea, tachycardia and pallor occur as with any chronic anaemia.
2. Glossitis, dysphagia and koilonychia are common features in nutritional deficiencies and are frequently seen in elderly people living alone.
3. In some cases dysphagia predominates and may simulate high oesophageal carcinoma.
4. Slight or moderate splenic enlargement may be found in any anaemia and cannot be considered specific.

Diagnosis

Points to note are:

1. Past history of indigestion, diarrhoea or black stools.
2. Menstrual history in women.
3. Intake of food, alcohol or drugs.
4. Examination for
   (a) bruising, petechiae, spider naevi in the skin
   (b) tenderness or mass in the abdomen
   (c) abnormality in rectum.

Investigations

1. Blood loss may be obvious. If not, chemical examination of the stools for occult blood will be positive. In cases of doubt, the test should be repeated after the patient has been on a meat-free diet for 72 hours.
2. Serum folate and serum B_{12} levels will indicate deficiency. A Schilling test will confirm impaired B_{12} absorption.
3. Proctoscopy and sigmoidoscopy should be carried out in all cases.
4. Barium meal and follow-through X-rays will show anatomical lesions as far as the ileo-caecal valve and in small gut malabsorption may give a typical pattern (flocculation and dilatation).
5. Double contrast Barium enema X-rays will demonstrate colonic tumours and ulceration.
6. Gastroscopy may be the only method of demonstrating gastric erosions or telangiectasia.

Treatment

1 **Iron**

The intestinal mucosa in health only permits the transference of up to 4 mgms. of food iron per day, a restriction which prevents the development of iron overload, there being no significant pathway for excretion of iron.

In iron deficiency states however the amount of iron absorbed through otherwise normal mucosa is increased in proportion to the depletion of body stores.

One standard 300 mgms. (5 grain) tablet of ferrous sulphate containing 40 mgms. of iron if absorbed completely raises the haemoglobin level at the maximum rate of 1% per day, but in practise patients are advised to take up to six such tablets daily, containing 240 mgms. of iron, to overcome variability in the absorption with different diets.

Many patients claim intolerance to oral iron which can cause colic, constipation or diarrhoea. The reaction is usually quantitative and smaller doses can often be well tolerated.

The treatment of iron deficiency anaemia should be continued for months rather than weeks. A number of the so-called iron-resistant anaemias are due to a failure on the part of the patient to take what has been prescribed.

2 **Hydroxycobalamin (Vitamin B_{12})**

This should always be given parenterally. Although a small quantity can be absorbed by the intestine in the absence of the intrinsic factor, this is unreliable. Inadequate Vitamin B_{12} replacement may allow the neurological complication of subacute combined degeneration of the cord to arise.

Immediate treatment of deficiency requires intramuscular injection of 5,000 to 10,000 μgms. in the first few weeks but subsequent maintenance needs are usually no more than 250 μgms. monthly of hydroxycobalamin.

3 **Folic acid**

This is well tolerated by mouth and a dose of 5 mgms. three times a day is adequate. When there is extensive abnormality of the intestinal mucosa, a folic acid preparation may need to be given parenterally.

CHAPTER 12

INTESTINAL INFECTIONS

Four separate groups of infecting agents are considered here, of which the bacteria are the most important.

'Gastroenteritis in infancy' is considered under a separate heading at the end of the chapter.

Classification
1 **Bacteria**
    - (a) **'Food poisoning'**
        - (i) **infective (salmonella etc.)**
        - (ii) **toxic (staphylococci etc.).**
    - (b) **Typhoid and paratyphoid**
    - (c) **Cholera**
    - (d) **Bacillary dysentery**
2 **Protozoa**
    - (a) **Amoebic dysentery**
    - (b) **Giardiasis**
3 **Viruses**
4 **Fungi**

Gastroenteritis in infancy.

1 BACTERIAL INFECTIONS

The bowel harbours a great variety of organisms living as commensals within the lumen which only cause disease under unusual circumstances. Many other varieties of bacteria however if introduced into the gut attack the mucous membrane of the bowel and some are dangerously pathogenic.

The majority gain access to the blood stream giving rise to systemic symptoms of toxaemia as well as causing local irrita-

Intestinal Infections 107

tion of the bowel wall which results in vomiting, colic and diarrhoea. Whether vomiting or diarrhoea is the predominant symptom depends largely on whether the upper or lower bowel is mainly involved in the infection and it is interesting that different types of bacteria attack different sections of the bowel. The dysentery organisms for instance have to pass through the length of the jejunum and ileum before arriving in a position to attack the colonic mucous membrane and yet they leave the small bowel untouched.

Most organisms confine their activities to the surface mucous membrane but some, classically the typhoid bacillus, concentrate in lymphoid tissue giving rise to inflammation of the Peyer's patches. Others again involve the whole thickness of the bowel wall and form a proliferative mass (e.g. tuberculosis). It is therefore hardly surprising that there are considerable differences in the clinical picture resulting from infection by the different organisms. Yet essentially these differences are merely variations in the degree of abdominal discomfort, vomiting, diarrhoea, malaise and fever.

(a) Food poisoning

Aetiology

All intestinal infections might be designated as food poisoning since the organisms gain entrance via food. However, common usage has limited the use of this term to certain groups of bacteria:

Salmonella (excluding Salm. typhosum and paratyphosum)
Staphylococci, streptococci
Clostridia

Food may be contaminated
  (i) before packing or carrying (e.g. dried egg powder and canned meats)
  (ii) in larders or kitchens where there is inadequate hygiene (e.g. trays of cold meats)

A distinction is sometimes drawn between 'infective' and 'toxic' food poisoning and although the separation is not complete, it is not without clinical significance.

In infective food poisoning the organisms have to proliferate within the intestine whereas in the toxic type they have already established themselves in the food and pre-formed toxins are present for immediate absorption.

Clinical features

(i) 'infective' food poisoning (mainly salmonella).

A time interval of 12 to 48 hours between ingestion and the development of symptoms is usual. The attack is concentrated upon the small bowel but the intensity of the inflammatory response and therefore the severity of the clinical picture varies considerably. Diarrhoea is the predominant feature.

The great majority of salmonella infections are mild but that due to salmonella typhimurium can be dangerously severe and occasionally is rapidly fatal.

(ii) 'toxic' food poisoning (mainly staphylococci, streptococci and clostridia).

Local and systemic symptoms are immediate as absorption of the preformed toxin is rapid but subsequently the course is the same as the organisms continue to proliferate in the bowel. Vomiting frequently occurs in the early stages.

In the case of infection with Clostridium Botulinum (Botulism) the toxin formed attacks nerve tissue so that neurological symptoms predominate. These include acute encephalitis, cranial nerve palsies and respiratory paralysis.

Investigations

1 Stool cultures may grow the causative organism.
2 Bacteriological culture of infective food (if any remains) may show contamination.
3 The source of contamination should be determined whereever possible to prevent further outbreaks of food poisoning.

Treatment

1 The simple salmonella organisms respond satisfactorily to sulphonamides which are best prescribed in a non-absorbable form so that higher concentrations can be achieved within the lumen of the bowel. Sulphasuxidine or sulphaphthalidine are the two most widely favoured. A loading

Intestinal Infections

dose of 4 gm. should be followed by 2 gm. q.d.s. for three or four days. Oral streptomycin is also very effective and is usefully combined with one of the sulphonamides.

2 Neomycin is more rapidly effective but has an adverse influence upon small intestinal absorption and occasionally will produce clinical steatorrheoa.

3 In very mild cases of non-specific food poisoning the iodine-containing hydroxyquinolines such as Enterovioform are adequate and have an advantage in that they do not mask the clinical picture, should a more specific organism be responsible.

4 Any of the above regimes should be accompanied by a simple diet and lessened activity. Fluid intake should be increased to compensate for the increased loss in the stool.

Staphylococcal Enterocolitis

Aetiology

This is due to infection with the staphylococcus aureus and merits special attention as it may be exceedingly dangerous. It can arise from the over-enthusiastic administration of a broad-spectrum antibiotic which suppresses the normal intestinal flora as well as destroying pathogens. The resulting 'sterile' bowel then becomes colonised by resistant organisms which are frequently of above average virulence.

Clinical features

Vomiting, diarrhoea and prostration are intense and of rapid onset. Deaths within 48 hours have been recorded. The mucosal lining may be stripped and when this occurs the description phlegmonous or 'pseudo-membranous' enterocolitis is sometimes used.

Investigations

1 Gram film of faeces may show an excess of staphylococci.
2 Culture on salt agar will enable staphylococci to be isolated.

Treatment

The situation demands urgent rehydration, measures to counter

110   *Lecture Notes on Gastroenterology*

shock (intravenous fluid—plasma or blood) and parenteral adminstration of large doses of Methicillin (Celbenin) 1 gm. 4—6 hourly. Supplementary steroids (100 mgm. hydrocortisone i.v.) are also indicated.

(b) Typhoid

Aetiology

This is an acute infection due to Salmonella typhosum occurring after the ingestion of faecally contaminated food or drink. Spread can occur from the faeces of healthy carriers or infected persons where hygiene is inadequate.

Pathology

The organisms initially are confined to the lymphoid tissue of the small intestine (Peyer's patches) but quickly spread to the blood stream and from there to the reticulo-endothelial system. Profuse growth may occur in the biliary tract and further organisms thus enter the gut.

It is not until the third week that the local inflammatory reaction in the bowel reaches its height when haemorrhage and perforation are liable to occur.

Clinical features

These are variable depending on the severity of the illness which is usually subacute in onset but which may be mild or at times overwhelming.

1. Systemic manifestations are fever, headache and toxaemia due to bacteraemia.
2. Local symptoms are abdominal colic and constipation at first, followed by abdominal tenderness and diarrhoea from the second week onwards.
3. Splenomegaly and a rose spot skin rash may be seen on abdominal examination.
4. The pulse is slow in relation to the degree of fever.
5. Extraintestinal complications such as pneumonitis, myocarditis, meningitis and osteitis may be present.

Investigations

1. Stool culture will demonstrate the organisms from the

fourth week onwards.
2 Blood culture will usually grow the organisms in the first week but becomes progressively less helpful thereafter.
3 The total white cell count tends to be low with a polymorphonuclear leucopaenia after the second week.
4 Widal serological reaction. Very high or rising titres are diagnostic.

Treatment

1 Bed rest and nursing care should be instituted as early as possible in the invasive stage, before the patient has become overtly ill.
2 Chemotherapy is also urgent and Chloramphenicol remains the drug of choice in spite of the potential risk of granulopaenia. In severe cases Chloramphenicol should be given in doses of 1 gm. six-hourly for three days, subsequently continuing with 0.5 gm. q.d.s. for at least a further week before reducing to the more usual level of 0.25 gm. six-hourly. This dose may then be required to be maintained for a month or more.

Ampicillin has been shown to be effective but its action is less rapid and subsequent relapse is more frequent.
3 Diet should be light but of high caloric value in order to enable the patient to combat the more serious toxic phase which usually develops during the second and third week.

Paratyphoid

Aetiology

This is due to Salmonella paratyphosum A or B and is usually a much less serious condition although some cases can be severe.

Clinical features

Abdominal discomfort and diarrhoea appear much earlier than in typhoid and are frequently the presenting symptom.

Investigations

As for typhoid.

Treatment

Being a less hazardous infection it is justifiable to avoid the use of Chloramphenicol and in its place to employ either Tetracycline or Ampicillin. Dosage is 500 mgm six-hourly for the first few days and subsequently 250 mgm q.d.s. for a week after the symptoms have been controlled.

(c) Cholera

Aetiology

This disease is due to the Vibrio cholerae and occurs most commonly in Asia. Infection is spread by contamination of water or food with infected faeces.

Pathology

The Vibrio cholerae is a particularly virulent organism which multiplies profusely within the lumen of the bowel. It attacks the mucous membrane giving rise to an acute inflammatory reaction.

Clinical features

1. The clinical picture is almostly exclusively the result of profound fluid and electrolyte loss.
   The incubation period may be no more than hours and the onset of the symptoms (diarrhoea, shock and dehydration) can be dramatically sudden. Death can result within a few days.
2. Diarrhoea may be profuse, the faeces resembling 'rice-water'.
3. Bleeding is only rarely evident.

Investigations

1. Microscopy of the stool often shows the vibrios in masses.
2. Stool culture will demonstrate the organism.

Treatment

The one urgent and over-riding essential is intravenous fluid replacement. 2—4 litres may be required in the first hour, alternating normal and half normal dextrose saline. Addition of

Intestinal Infections 113

potassium may also be required but this must be given with care.

Antibiotics are of limited value, more especially since they have to be given orally in order to inhibit the intra-luminal proliferation of the vibrio. This may be difficult or impossible to achieve during vomiting. The non-absorbable sulphonamides are probably best but Chloromycetin, Tetracycline. Streptomycin and Neomycin are all said to be active against the vibrio.

(d) Bacillary dysentery

Aetiology

This results from infection by the Shigella group of organisms. Sh. shiga is the most virulent member of the group. Sh. sonnei is relatively benign and is responsible for most of the mild examples of this illness.

Pathology

The infection primarily involves the colon but may also affect the small bowel. There is localised inflammation with oedema and superficial ulceration. Perforation is rare.

Clinical features

1. The condition has an incubation period of 1—7 days.
2. The symptoms vary from mild diarrhoea to an acute fulminating illness with generalised abdominal pain, tenesmus, incontinence of heavily bloodstained stools and severe toxaemia.
3. A less definite relapsing variety can occur but only rarely is a case of chronic bacillary dysentery encountered.

Investigations

1. Stool culture may demonstrate the causative organism.
2. A blood count will show a polymorphonuclear leucocytosis.

Treatment

This consists of:
1. Bed rest.
2. Fluid replacement.

114 *Lecture Notes on Gastroenterology*

Fluids can usually be given by mouth but in the more severe cases the intravenous route may be necessary. Sufficient volume should be given to maintain a urinary output of over one litre and if diarrhoea is profuse, electrolyte replacement will also be needed.

3 Chemotherapy.

The agent of choice is oxytetracycline (1.0 gm. initially followed by 0.5 gm. four-hourly). Although the sulphonamides are effective against shigella organisms, the non-absorbable varieties (sulphasuccidine and sulphathalidine) may not act quickly enough. In tropical climates the use of the soluble varieties (sulphadiazine or sulphathiazole) is not advisable owing to the risk of crystalluria.

2 PROTOZOAL INFECTIONS

(a) Amoebic Dysentery

Aetiology

This is an infection primarily involving the colon and due to invasion of the mucosa by Entamoeba histolytica. It is more common in tropical climates. It arises from the contamination of food or water with faeces containing amoebic cysts.

Pathology

The walls of the ingested cysts are broken down by digestive enzymes in the gut lumen thus releasing motile amoebic trophozoites (amoebae). The amoebae may gain access to the liver via the portal venous system and there give rise to a focal hepatitis which later may progress to abscess formation.

Clinical features

1 The condition is nearly always more protracted than bacillary dysentery although an acute form is occasionally encountered.
2 The patient experiences recurrent episodes of diarrhoea and the bowels are opened approximately six to twelve times daily.
3 The stools may be bloodstained the mucoid element predominates.

Intestinal Infections 115

4 There may be little or no abdominal discomfort and fever is unusual.

Investigation

1 Examination of a warm fresh stool is essential if trophozoites are to be found.
2 Sigmoidoscopy may reveal the ulcers and cysts found in rectal biopsy specimens.

Treatment

This must be thorough to avoid recurrence.
1 For gut involvement: Emetine hydrochloride remains the agent of choice in the intial stages in spite of its undeniably toxic effect on the myocardium. Because of the risk of heart failure, full bed rest is obligatory during the four to ten day (according to the severity) course of 60 mg. daily intramuscularly. Emetine will deal with any active amoebae in the bowel wall or tissues but must be followed up by a prolonged oral course of an iodine-containing compound to maintain an amoebicidal environment within the lumen of the bowel e.g. Emetine bismuth iodide 60 mgms. t.d.s. Each dose should be given with food and preceded by 30—60 mgms. of Phenobarbitone or 25 mgms. Avomine to suppress the nausea.

Subsequently di-iodohydroxyquinoline (Embequin) should be given in doses of 300 mgms. t.d.s. for at least three weeks.

Tetracycline is amoebicidal but is insufficiently reliable for sole use. The same is possibly true of the newer agent Paranomycin (Humatin). Neither control hepatic amoebiasis.

2 For liver involvement: The initial parenteral course of Emetine hydrochloride should be followed by Chloroquin which concentrates a hundredfold within the liver. The dosage is 250 mgms. t.d.s. for two weeks.

(b) Giardiasis (Giardia lamblia)

Aetiology

Infection of the small intestine with Giardia lamblia may

occur on its own or in association with E. histolytica infection. It is common in tropical countries and in areas where hygiene and nutrition are poor.

Pathology
1 Trophozoites can be found in the lumen of the bowel and also on or in the mucosa.
2 The small intestinal mucosa may show blunting of the villi and an increased cellular infiltrate.
   These changes are reversible.

Clinical features
The majority of infective persons are without symptoms but there may be:
1 Diarrhoea, which is usually mild but can be surprisingly severe.
2 Vomiting and abdominal discomfort.
3 A malabsorption syndrome.

Investigations
1 Microscopic examination of faeces will demonstrate cysts or trophozoites of giardia. Further faecal studies should be carried out after treatment to exclude an underlying E. histolytica infection.
2 Duodenal aspiration may contain trophozoites.
3 Jejunal biopsy may show morphological changes.
4 A Barium follow-through may demonstrate a malabsorption pattern.

Treatment
Quinacrine (Atabrine) in a dosage of 0.1 gm. t.d.s. for five days is successful in almost all cases.

3 VIRUS INFECTIONS

Aetiology
Many of the mild episodes of gastroenteritis which affect the community are undoubtedly of virus origin but in the absence of specific tests the diagnosis can only be presumptive.

Pathology

Whether or not the virus is specifically pathogenic to the intestinal mucosa or whether the diarrhoea and vomiting are merely an expression of a generalised infection is open to debate. Little is known of the histological changes in the mucosa owing to the mild nature of the disorder.

Clinical features

1. The commonest presentation is that of a shortlived, 24—72 hour, illness with vomiting and diarrhoea associated with low-grade fever, generalised aches and abdominal tenderness.
2. It is frequently met with in localised epidemics.
3. Fortunately the disease is selflimiting but is often followed by a protracted convalescent phase of malaise and emotional depression.

Investigations

1. Isolation of the organism on viral culture from stool specimens is not yet possible in most cases.
2. Serial serological examination at 0, 2 and 6 weeks may help in the retrospective epidemiological study of some outbreaks.

Treatment

This consists of:
1. Rest, light diet and plenty of fluids.
2. Relief of symptoms with antiemetics and antidiarrhoeal agents.

4 FUNGUS INFECTIONS

Aetiology

Candida albicans (moniliasis) is the commonest agent and the usual underlying cause is the prolonged administration of broad spectrum antibiotics. Spontaneous establishment of these organisms rarely occurs on account of the presence of the saprophytic bacteria.

Pathology

The infection occurs most commonly in the mouth and may spread to involve the bowel or the lungs. It is more common in the severely ill and those with a dry mouth.

Clinical features

1. Sore tongue, diarrhoea and pruritis ani are common and may be exceedingly persistent.
2. Patches of white exudate may be seen on the mouth and pharynx ('thrush').

Investigations

1. Bacterial examination of a throat swab may demonstrate the organisms.
2. Stool examination may also show the organisms.

Treatment

This consists of:
1. Specific treatment with
   (a) Nystatin 1,000,000 units q.d.s. in tablet form to combat the gut infection
   (b) Nystatin in solution (200,000 units per ml.) as mouth-washes for the mouth infection
   (c) Nystatin suppositories (100,000 units) for the rectal infection.
2. Re-establishment of a normal intestinal bacterial population
   (a) By withdrawal of other antibiotics where practicable
   (b) By administration of lactobacilli or other faecal flora in capsule form.
3. Supplemental vitamin B. This is sometimes given in the belief that vitamin B absorption is less with altered intestinal flora. Frank vitamin deficiencies are not seen.

GASTRO-ENTERITIS IN INFANCY

Causes

1. Infective diarrhoea due to:
   Bact. coli

Intestinal Infections 119

Viruses (non-specific)
Dysenteric organisms, most commonly Shigella Sonnei.
2 Dietetic diarrhoea, rarely serious or prolonged.
3 Symptomatic diarrhoea i.e. that associated with infections outside the alimentary tract e.g. otitis media, urinary infections. In the early months of life, Group 1 is the commonest cause. Sonnei infection usually affects older infants and toddlers and is betrayed by the presence of blood and mucus in the stools.

'D & V' is always a serious disease in infants because of their immature immunological response and their labile biochemical balance.

Clinical features

The symptoms in the form of loose, frequent, green watery stools often appear almost explosively and the infant very rapidly shows clinical and biochemical evidence of severe dehydration.

Investigations

Stool culture may demonstrate the causative organism.

Treatment

1 This consists of immediate restoration of the fluid and electrolyte balance, usually by intravenous drip and expert nursing is essential.
2 Chemotherapy and antibiotic therapy is disappointing and cannot be relied upon alone.
3 Isolation of children infected in institutions i.e. nurseries and hospitals is urgent in order to prevent epidemics.

Prognosis

In tropical countries gastro-enteritis is the chief killing infection in infancy but in the U.K. the severity and frequency has lessened to a remarkable degree due to better infant hygiene with better knowledge of electrolyte control. As so often happens the younger the baby the more severe the disease is likely to be.

CHAPTER 13

HELMINTH INFESTATIONS

Classification
1 **Cestodes**
2 **Nematodes**
3 **Trematodes**

1 CESTODES

There are four common tapeworms known to infest man, three of which have their adult existence within the lumen of the human intestine while the fourth establishes itself in the cystic stage in his tissues.
 (a) Taenia saginata
 (b) Taenia solium
 (c) Dibothriocephalus latus
 (d) Taenia echinococcus.

(a) Taenia Saginata (beef tapeworm)
Herbivorous animals (cattle, sheep, giraffes, llamas and buffaloes) are the intermediate hosts for this worm which can attain considerable length when fully developed in its human host (10—15 feet). The segments are enlongated and may number as many as 1,500. They increase in size as they mature. The tiny head (scolex) carries four suckers but no hooklets.

(b) Taenia Solium (pork tapeworm)
The chief difference between this variety which has the pig as its intermediate host and the other tapeworms is the head which possesses a double row of hooklets in addition to the four suckers.

(c) Dibothriocephalus Latus (fish tapeworm)

The segments of this worm are broad and it attains the greatest length of all the human tapeworms. Fish are the intermediate hosts.

Clinical features

These worms usually occur singly and usually the sole indication of their presence is the intermittent passage of segments (proglottides) in the stool. Only in the rare instances of heavy infestation or in persons of borderline nutrition are there any clinical manifestations in the form of malaise and weight loss.

Infestation with dibothriocephalus latus may give rise to a macrocytic anaemia due to the fact that this worm competes for the small available supplies of B_{12} in the intestine.

Diagnosis

Examination of freshly passed faeces will demonstrate the detached segments.

Treatment

1 Quinacrine hydrochloride (Atabrin, Mepacrin) is the simplest and safest agent for the eradication of all three types of tapeworm. There are certain difficulties in administration as it is nauseating and it is important to avoid vomiting lest any of the proglottides be inhaled into the lung, since this enables the cystic stage to become established in man (cysticercosis).

The following régime is advocated:
   (a) A light fluid diet only on the previous few days.
   (b) A saline purge on the preceding evening.
   (c) A sedative anti-emetic on waking (Phenobarbitone 60 mgms., Chlorpromazine 50 mgms., or Avomine 25 mgms.)
   (d) One hour later two 100 mgm. tablets or quinacrine hydrochloride which dose is repeated five times at five minute intervals (total 1 gm.).
   (e) Two hours later a generous saline purge.
   (f) Stools are preserved and sieved through black muslin in order to identify the scolex.

If such therapy is ineffective it may be repeated one week later.

A more certain method is to adminster the quinacrine hydrochloride down an indwelling duodenal tube.

2 In refractory cases resort may have to be made to the more toxic agent, Felix Mas, and for this the following additional precautions are advisable:
   (a) Dietary fat should be excluded for 48 hours and the patient subjected to complete starvation for 24 hours preceding therapy. Subsequently all food should be withheld until after successful purgation has been achieved.
   (b) Preliminary sedative anti-emetic medication is advisable as above and the Felix Mas is given in divided doses of 2 ml. at five minute intervals up to a maximum of 8 ml.

(d) Taenia Echinococcus

In this instance the adult worm resides in the animal (dog) host. It is very small (2—6 mm.) and consists of a head and three segments only.

Human infection results from ingestion of the eggs. After hatching the larvae penetrate the duodenal wall and are dispersed throughout the body. Although, as might be expected, the liver is the main site of lodgement and subsequent development, any organ may be involved. Hydatid cysts may attain great dimensions and take many years to mature.

The disease is commonest in sheep farming communities—in Australia and South Africa, but its distribution is worldwide and the disease can be acquired in the British Isles.

Clinical features

The cysts may present:
1 Due to their clinical size, presenting as tumours.
2 Occasionally secondary infections supervene, in which case local pain, fever and leucocytosis will result.
3 The cyst may rupture and evoke a dangerously acute allergic response with asthma and urticaria.
4 As a chance finding as a calcified cyst on radiography.
5 Eosinophilia is an inconstant finding in uncomplicated cases.

Diagnosis

The Casoni test utilises active hydatid fluid as an antigen and a 5 cm. weal may be expected to appear in positive cases within twenty minutes of the 0.2 ml. intradermal injection.

A variety of other immunological tests have been elaborated but are less universally available.

Treatment

1. No immediate treatment may be required for an asymptomatic calcified cyst in the liver but the patient should be kept under review.
2. In other cases treatment is surgical removal if possible. The greatest care has to be taken to avoid rupture of the cyst during the procedure since not only is an allergic reaction likely but the disease may be disseminated by seeding of the daughter cysts.

2 NEMATODES

Disease	Worm
(a) Ankylostomiasis (hookworm)	Ankylostoma duodenale Necator Americanus
(b) Enterobiasis (threadworm)	Enterobius (oxyuris) vermicularis
(c) Ascariasis (roundworm)	Ascaris lumbricoides
(d) Strongyloidiasis	Strongyloides stercoralis
(e) Trichuriasis (whipworm)	Trichuris trichiura
(f) Trichinosis	Trichinella spiralis

(a) Ankylostomiasis (hookworm)

The Ankylostoma duodenale and Necator Americanus inhabit the upper part of the small intestine. The worm is small, only some 8—13 mm. in length, but may be present in very large numbers. It hangs on to the mucous membrane by means of clawed teeth and subsists by absorbing blood from its human host.

The life cycle of these two worms in interesting. The female lays eggs in the small intestine which are passed in the stool. These eggs hatch in the soil and develop into infective larvae. On contact with the skin of the human host, they penetrate and are carried via the blood stream to the lungs. They enter the bronchial tree via the alveoli and ascend to pass over the epiglottis and so down the oesophagus to reach the small intestine.

Clinical features

When infestation is heavy, symptoms are those of anaemia due to blood loss. Abdominal discomfort is uncommon. Even in less severe cases the stool will show a consistently positive test for occult blood and the differential white cell count may reveal the presence of an eosinophilia.

Diagnosis

This depends upon the demonstration of the characteristic eggs in the stool, the numbers of which also give some guide as to the degree of infestation. Local skin irritation may be noted at the point of entry and exceptionally there are transient pulmonary symptoms, such as cough or even haemoptysis.

Treatment

Bephenium naphthoate (Alcopar) has the great merit of low toxicity and can therefore be used with safety even in severely anaemic and debilitated patients. A single dose of 1.25—2.25 g. according to body weight is often adequate but successive administration for up to three days is claimed to be without risk. Tetrachlorethylene may be necessary for resistant cases in doses of 2.0—4.0 ml., preceded and followed by a mild saline purge. In addition to anthelmintics, haematinics are obviously indicated for the anaemia. Iron is essential but both folic acid and B_{12} may be needed in severely depleted cases.

(b) Enterobiasis (threadworm)

This is a very common infection in both adults and children. The worm is small and white, approximately 10 mm. long and inhabits the region of the caecum.

Clinical features

The characteristic symptom of anal pruritus is caused by migra-

Helminth Infestations

tion of the females through the sphincter for the purpose of laying eggs.

Diagnosis

The ova can be demonstrated microscopically by examination of cellophane perianal swabs or transparent adhesive tape strips which have been pressed against the anal area.

Treatment

Dissemination from one member of the family to another is the usual course and treatment should be administered to all simultaneously.

Piperazine citrate (Antepar) is the agent of choice and is given in a seven day course (50—75 mg./kg. daily). Gentian violet gr. 1 t.d.s. is equally effective but inordinately messy.

(c) Ascariasis (roundworm)

Second only to the threadworm, the ascaris is the most frequently encountered nematode in a temperate climate. It bears close resemblance to the common earth worm although it is somewhat more tapered at both ends.

Ascarids, like tapeworms, often exist singly in adult patients. In children, however, multiple infestation is frequent and the worm population can be so profuse as to cause intestinal obstruction.

Clinical features

The ascaris usually gives little indication of its presence. Occasionally the worm can migrate back into the stomach and may appear as a constituent of the vomit.

A transient pneumonia may signal the invasive stage as after hatching the larvae migrate via the mesenteric lymphatics or portal vein, through the right heart to the lungs. Subsequently they find their way back down into the alimentary canal by way of the trachea and oesophagus.

Diagnosis

If the worm is passed in the stool or appears in the vomit, the diagnosis is obvious, but more usually this has to depend upon identification of the characteristic eggs in the stool.

The presence of an eosinophilia in association with pulmonary symptoms is suggestive of ascaris pneumonitis but eosinophilia is less consistently associated with simple intestinal infection.

Treatment

Piperazine has the merit of being simple, safe and effective and is in addition well tolerated by the patient. It does not require any preliminary preparation and a single dose is usually adequate. The citrate, adipate or phosphate salts are equally suitable since they all form piperazine hexahydrate in solution. The ascaris is only paralysed by piperazine and whereas this reduces the risk of sensitivity reactions occurring as a consequence of toxic absorption from destroyed dead worms, it necessitates the subsequent use of a saline purge to flush the parasite from the intestinal lumen. Dose: 150 mg./kg. body weight piperazine citrate which, if necessary, can be repeated one week later.

Other equally effective agents for ascariasis are Bephenium, Diathiazine and Hexyl Resorcinol.

(d), (e) Strongyloidiasis and Trichuriasis

The strongyloides is relatively small (0.5—2 mm.) and the trichuria slightly larger (3—5 cm.). This latter has a long flagella-like tail, hence its designation whip worm.

Clinical features

These two nematodes are of lesser importance since they rarely cause significant bowel symptoms.

Diagnosis

The worms or their ova can be demonstrated in freshly passed faeces.

Treatment

Diathiazine iodine (Telmid) was the drug of choice but recently some doubts have been raised as to its safety. However both Bephenium and pierazine are also effective.

Dosage of diathiazine: 100 mg. t.d.s. A course of 2—3 weeks is preferable.

(f) Trichinosis (trichinella spiralis)

This is fortunately a relatively rare infestation in which the cystic stage takes place in man.

Man contracts the condition from eating infested pork. The small worms hatch in the upper intestine and mate before the female penetrates the mucous membrane to deposit her larvae. These are then distributed by the blood stream to all parts of the body where they embed themselves in muscle tissue.

Clinical features

During the invasive phase myalgic pains and fever occur and an eosinophilia is produced. Periorbital swelling is a specific feature but oedema is not confined to the face. Salivary glands may be enlarged and a scarlatiniform rash appears. In severe cases there may be dyspnoea and even evidence of myocarditis with failure.

Diagnosis

1 Muscle biopsy in suspected cases may reveal the larvae or cysts.
2 Intradermal skin testing with trichinella antigen may be helpful.

Treatment

Until recently no specific agent has been available for any of the tissue-invading nematodes. Thiabadazole, a chemical related to Vitamin B_{12} has recently been introduced and may possibly be effective in the invasive stages in doses of 50 mg./kg. for two days.

3 TREMATODES

Biharziasis (intestinal schistosomiasis)

One variety of this parasite (S. Mansoni) infests the mesenteric veins and gives rise to gastrointestinal symptoms. In the later stage the liver is invaded with the eventual production of cirrhosis.

Water snails are the intermediate hosts and the parasite gains entrance to the human through the unbroken skin, hence the danger of bathing or walking in infested waters. The cercariae enter the circulation and are carried to the lungs, subsequently being distributed to all parts of the body. They finally establish themselves in the portal veins where they develop into adult forms. After mating they migrate distally into the mesenteric veins, especially the haemorrhoidal plexuses and lay their eggs in the venules of the intestinal mucosa.

Clinical features

The invasive stage may be asymptomatic but on the other hand general toxaemia may be severe with fever, rigors, nausea, vomiting and diarrhoea. There may also be urticaria or even extensive angioneurotic oedema.

The infiltrative stage manifests itself any time between two and twenty-four months later. The dominant symptoms are then abdominal colic and diarrhoea. The stool contains blood and mucus.

In the heavily infested case there is general body wasting, hepato-splenomegaly and a remittant fever. Occasionally the thickened colon or enlarged mesenteric nodes may be felt.

In a few cases both the invasive and the infiltrative phases may pass unnoticed and the patient presents with the symptoms of portal hypertension due to hepatic cirrhosis.

Diagnosis

Microscopic examination of the faeces reveals the characteristic lateral spined eggs of the parasite.

Treatment

Schistosomiasis is a most refractory condition and for the course of the disease to be influenced, intensive therapy is necessary. The choice of drug is still controversial since all preparations are highly toxic.

The two most frequently employed drugs are potassium antimony tartrate (tartar emetic) and antimony pyrocatechin disulfonate (stibophen). The former has to be given intravenously but the latter can be administered intramuscularly. Administration must be progressive and prolonged and the maximum care taken to guard against myocardial toxicity. Full bed rest conditions and E.C.G. monitoring of the injections is advisable.

CHAPTER 14
DIARRHOEA

Definition

An increase in either frequency or fluidity of the stool is the generally accepted medical interpretation of diarrhoea. However since the range of normality in the pattern of bowel activity is variable and since the term is all too often loosely used, it is essential to obtain a detailed description of what each individual patient means when he complains of diarrhoea.

Classification of causes
1 **Infections**
   - **(a) Bacterial**
   - **(b) Protozoal**
   - **(c) Viral**
   - **(d) Fungal**
   - **(e) Parasitic**
2 **Irritants**
   - **(a) Bacterial (toxins)**
   - **(b) Chemical (poisons)**
   - **(c) Drugs**
   - **(d) Radiation**
3 **Digestive secretion defects**
   - **(a) Achlorhydria**
   - **(b) Pancreatic insufficiency**
4 **Absorptive faults**
   - **(a) Resected or short circuited bowel**
   - **(b) Blind loop syndrome**
   - **(c) Small intestinal diverticulosis**
   - **(d) Infiltrative disease of the bowel wall**
   - **(e) Gluten enteropathy or sprue**
   - **(f) Mucosal enzyme deficiencies**

5 Idiopathic inflammatory disease
        (a) **Regional enteritis**
        (b) **Ulcerative colitis**
6 Allergic reactions
        (a) **General**
        (b) **Local**
7 Vascular disturbances
        Mesenteric vascular occlusion—arterial, venous
8 Metabolic derangements
        (a) **Uraemia**
        (b) **Diabetes**
9 Endocrine dyscrasias
        (a) **Hyperthyroidism**
        (b) **Islet cell tumour of the pancreas (non-insulin secreting)**
10 Nervous influences
        (a) **Anxiety**
        (b) **Vagotomy**
        (c) **Diabetes**
11 Spurious diarrhoea
        (a) **Faecal impaction**
        (b) **Rectal tumours**
        (c) **Granular proctitis**

1 INFECTIONS

Although these are undoubtedly a frequent cause of diarrhoea, they are by no means the only aetiological factor. They are discussed in detail in Chapter 12.

2 IRRITANTS

Diarrhoea may result from the presence of irritants in the small or large bowel. These irritants may be formed in the gut or be introduced accidentally or therapeutically.

(a) Bacterial

Occasionally irritant 'toxins' are the products of bacterial activity, e.g. bacillus botulinus and certain other anaerobic organisms.

(b) Chemical

Chemical agents such as arsenicals and mercurials, may cause diarrhoea.

On the other hand some poisons give rise to constipation, e.g. lead poisoning.

(c) Drugs

The aperients are all too frequently overlooked as a cause of diarrhoea. Over-enthusiastic self-medication is very common and is often carried out owing to the conviction that sluggish bowel activity is injurious to health.

Many other drugs have an irritant effect on the bowel and although symptoms such as nausea or vomiting usually appear first, diarrhoea may dominate the clinical picture. Digitalis, colchicine and quinidine are among the commonest agents and to these the anticoagulants and anti-hypertensive drugs must be added.

Broad spectrum antibiotics are sometimes responsible for a troublesome diarrhoea due to alteration of the bowel flora. Neomycin has a direct effect on the small intestinal mucosa and produces steatorrhoea by interfering with absorption.

(d) Radiation

Radiation is another cause of diarrhoea and this may prove to be a limiting factor when treating abdominal malignancies by deep X-ray.

3 DIGESTIVE SECRETION DEFECTS

(a) Achlorhydria (achylia gastrica)

Formerly it was thought that diminution or absence of gastric juice could be responsible for diarrhoea (lienteric diarrhoea) and regular medication with hydrochloric acid was prescribed. Were this concept entirely true, then all cases of pernicious anaemia should exhibit the symptoms of diarrhoea.

While it is now recognised that neither hydrochloric acid nor pepsin are indispensable for satisfactory digestive activity, it has to be remembered that gastric acid is highly bacteriocidal and serves as an effective first line defence against the entry of intestinal pathogens. In its absence there is a higher theoretical risk of infective food poisoning.

(b) Pancreatic insufficiency

If there is an insufficient secretion of pancreatic enzymes into the duodenum, normal digestion is incomplete and this results in intraluminal fermentation and diarrhoea due to irritation of the mucosa.

Such deficiency can occur as a result of diffuse pancreatic disease or of pancreatic duct obstruction.

(i) Diffuse disease

In practice diarrhoea due to this cause is relatively rare because even a reduced secretory volume is sufficient for basal digestive requirements.

In subacute relapsing pancreatitis the functional capacity of the gland is progressively impaired but the disorder may continue for years before diarrhoea or steatorrhoea become obvious.

Occasionally the pancreas may be entirely destroyed by acute pancreatitis and survivors of this condition are likely to suffer from diabetes and diarrhoea.

Carcinoma of the pancreas usually takes the form of a localised tumour and only occasionally is sufficiently diffuse to replace the whole gland, hence the relative rarity of diarrhoea due to this cause.

(ii) Duct obstruction

A gallstone impacted in the ampulla of Vater may obstruct the pancreatic duct as a result of local oedema and inflammation even when the biliary and pancreatic systems do not share a common terminal channel.

A carcinoma of the ampulla of Vater is another cause of obstruction to secretory flow and can result in the diagnostic triad of jaundice, steatorrhoea and occult blood in the stool. Diarrhoea may not be severe but the stools are usually unformed. When bleeding is consistent the stool may develop a characteristic silvery appearance due to a combination of the pallor of acholia and the black of melaena.

Benign and malignant tumours of the pancreas and sometimes fibrosis may cause obstruction to the main pancreatic duct.

4 ABSORPTIVE FAULTS

This subject is discussed more fully in Chapter 10 on Malabsorption Syndrome. Suffice it to say here that although steatorrhoea and diarrhoea are common features of the malabsorption syndrome, severe malabsorption can be present in the absence of diarrhoea.

5 IDIOPATHIC INFLAMMATORY CONDITIONS

Regional enterocolitis (Crohn's disease)
Ulcerative colitis

Both of these conditions are discussed more fully in their respective chapters but a few comments are appropriate here in relation to the problem of the differential diagnosis of diarrhoea. In ulcerative colitis the basic lesion is an inflammatory reaction exclusively confined to the mucosa of the large bowel and therefore diarrhoea is an almost invariable feature.

In regional enteritis the lesion is a granulomatous inflammatory reaction involving the whole thickness of the bowel wall. The small intestine is the site most commonly affected and consequently intermittent colic is a more consistent symptom than is diarrhoea. When the large intestine is involved, diarrhoea is more in evidence and it may be difficult, if not impossible, to distinguish it clinically from that due to ulcerative colitis.

6 ALLERGIC REACTIONS

(a) General

Diarrhoea may occasionally be a part of a severe generalised allergic reaction (anaphylactoid shock).

(b) Local

Considering the basic similarity between the intestinal and the nasal mucosa and also the high incidence of hay fever in the community, it is somewhat surprising to find that food allergies are relatively uncommon. However, that such allergies do exist is indisputable. When present it is usually singularly specific and the patient has long since made his own diagnosis. Oysters provide the classic example of a specific intestinal sensitivity response, but other shellfish can be highly provocative in certain individuals.

Other food sensitivities are of common occurrence and some cases of mild afebrile diarrhoea in people otherwise enjoying a 'Continental holiday' may well be instances of an allergic response. While it is impossible to prove that such cases are examples of mucosal allergy, the fact that many show a satisfactory response to mild antihistaminic agents and to small doses of codeine phosphate without antibiotics, is at least suggestive.

Milk protein is often stated to be a potential if not a frequent intestinal allergen and even has been said to be the cause of certain idiopathic diseases, such as regional enteritis and ulcerative colitis. However, although milk antibodies may be found in the serum of patients suffering from these two conditions, it is doubtful if milk is ever the primary cause.

Recent studies have revealed that even in those individuals in whom there is a consistent relationship between ingestion of milk and subsequent diarrhoea, the probability is that deficiency of the intramucosal enzyme lactase is the true cause of the bowel hyperactivity.

Coeliac disease may be included under the heading of allergy, since the causal relationship between the presence of wheat gluten and the mucosal changes has been well established, even though the exact mechanism involved remains incompletely understood. This condition is often referred to by the descriptive term gluten-induced enteropathy.

7 VASCULAR DISTURBANCES

Mesenteric vascular occlusion may be arterial or venous.

Symptoms (ill defined abdominal pain and diarrhoea) are similar in either instance but tend to be more severe in the arterial cases.

The diarrhoea is the result of bowel wall ischaemia and there is usually some accompanying blood loss. Depending upon the severity and the site of involvement this will appear either as melaena or frank haemorrhage.

It may be possible to obtain a preceding history of central abdominal pain following meals; the so-called 'abdominal angina' or 'chronic mid-gut ischaemia'.

8 METABOLIC DERANGEMENTS

(a) Uraemia

Even in advanced renal failure only a small number of patients develop diarrhoea but when present this symptom may be difficult to treat and is sometimes accompanied by a severe degree of bleeding.

Uraemic ulceration of both small and large bowel may be extensive and death may result from perforation. More usually the uraemic patient has moderate but overt looseness of stool.

(b) Diabetes

Diarrhoea in diabetes should be regarded as a complication rather than part of the symptom complex. The exact cause is unproven but it is possible that a neuropathy involving the autonomic nervous system may play a part and there is usually but not always an associated peripheral neuritis. Arteriopathy is another possible cause although frank mesenteric vascular occlusion is rare.

9 ENDOCRINE DYSCRASIAS

(a) Hyperthyroidism

Looseness of bowel activity is a common feature of overt thyrotoxicosis but it may occasionally be the presenting symptom and sometimes antedates the more common features of goitre, ner-

Diarrhoea 137

vous irritability, weight loss or eye signs.

The stool is usually watery but otherwise unremarkable. As might be expected, the bowel activity is often accentuated by stress, thus stimulating a simple anxiety response. Curiously enough, it rarely disturbs sleep at night.

(b) Islet cell tumours of the pancreas (non-insulin secreting)

This interesting rarity is more often present with intractable peptic ulceration than diarrhoea but the latter can be alarmingly severe and persistent. The diarrhoea results from both the irritation of the small intestine by massive gastric hypersecretion and the inactivation of the pancreatic enzymes by the altered pH.

10 NEUROLOGICAL INFLUENCES

(a) Anxiety

Emotion exerts its influence via the autonomic nervous pathways and is probably the commonest of all the many causes of diarrhoea. It is sometimes clearly related in time to the anxiety situation (e.g. academic examinations) but in the more chronic anxiety states it may be continuous and consequently the association is less obvious.

Such bowel hyperactivity is an increased physiological response and if a convincing explanation and adequate reassurance is forthcoming, the symptom responds to simple non-specific therapy, even when the causative background itself is incapable of resolution.

Mild basal sedation (Amylobarbitone 30 mgm. t.d.s.) is all that is necessary in the majority of instances, with the addition of a little Kaolin or Codein in the more refractory cases.

(b) Vagotomy

This procedure, accompanied by either pyloroplasty or gastroenterostomy, is becoming increasingly favoured as the surgical technique of choice in cases of recurrent or chronic duodenal ulcer. While the results as regards symptomatic relief and prevention of ulcer recurrence are excellent, a small percentage of cases subsequently develop diarrhoea.

In some degree, a change of bowel habits is almost invariable but in the majority of cases it amounts to no more than relief from previous constipation. It may be severe enough to cause inconvenience or in a few cases it may prove to be a considerable trial.

An explanation of post-vagotomy diarrhoea may possibly lie in the severance of the parasympathetic supply to the pancreas, resulting in reduced output of the exocrine secretion. For this reason selective vagotomy has been advocated, the aim of which is to preserve the coeliac branches of the vagus.

(c) Diabetes

The occasional association of diarrhoea with diabetes has been mentioned above and it has been proposed that it may result from a neuropathy involving the autonomic nerve supply to the intestine.

11 SPURIOUS DIARRHOEA

(a) Faecal impaction

This condition is frequently encountered in the aged who have lost the muscular power necessary for adequate defaecation. In consequence, a mass of faeces forms in the rectum and acts as a partially obstructive plug.

In the effort to overcome this the proximal bowel becomes overactive and its fluid plus mucus content is intermittently forced past the sides of the faecal impactation producing a clinical picture of diarrhoea. The weakened anal sphincter is rendered incompetent by the physical presence of the impacted mass, resulting in the additional distress of incontinence.

These patients can easily be relieved once the true situation has been recognised by a simple digital rectal examination.

(b) Rectal carcinoma

Low rectal cancers can produce a very similar clinical picture to that of faecal impaction but there is often haemorrhage as well, indicating that this is not a simple disorder.

Even when the tumour is higher in the bowel it may still present with the symptom of diarrhoea. This is especially so when it is a mucus-secreting type of growth.

Only later when partial obstruction is present does the classical alternation between constipation and diarrhoea develop.

(c) Granular proctitis

This condition is probably only a variant of ulcerative colitis, the inflammatory reaction being confined to the rectum for many years.

When the inflammation is acute, discharge of the serosanguinous exudate from the inflamed mucous membrane may give rise to the impression of diarrhoea. The patient often has a repeated urge to defaecate but passes no more than a little blood and mucus at each sitting.

DIFFERENTIAL DIAGNOSIS

History

As will have been appreciated from the foregoing, a careful history is of paramount importance in the differential diagnosis of diarrhoea. In many cases the cause can be confidently deduced from this alone.

Physical examination

This must be general as well as local. Abdominal palpation is often unhelpful but digital rectal examination is obligatory.

Sigmoidoscopy

This should be carried out in cases of diarrhoea before treatment where practicable and in all cases where symptoms persist in spite of treatment. Inflammatory disease of the rectum and distal tumours can be examined and mucosal swabs and biopsies taken through the instrument.

Personal inspection of a fresh stool

This is all too often evaded but it can be valuable in diagnosis and on occasions gives a complete answer to the problem.

Microscopy also gives a great deal of information and culture of the stool is essential.

X-ray studies

Barium X-ray studies have a valuable place in the differential diagnosis of diarrhoea and a Barium meal and follow-through as well as a Barium enema may be required to demonstrate disease in the small or large bowel.

TREATMENT

Apart from scientific measures directed at definitive causes, there are a few simple symptomatic remedies which can be employed to moderate the situation. In many cases this may be all that is necessary.

Kaolin is traditional and remains of great value. It is usually prescribed in combination with calcium carbonate (Mist. Kaolin B.P.C.). For greater efficacy a few minims of tinct. opii can be added (Mist.Kaolin sed. B.P.C.). Many proprietary preparations are available of similar constitution and with equivalent effect. Mist. Cret. Aromat. c Opio B.P.C. should be used with discretion in long-term cases for fear of initiating an addiction. In such patients, especially in colitis, Codeine Phosphate 30-60 mgms. two to four times daily is less hazardous and may be equally effective.

Belladonna and its derivatives are sometimes useful but the newer synthetic anticholinergics have little to offer over Atropine sulphate gr. 1/100 or Tinct. Bellad. m V—X in water three or four times daily. More recently various synthetic compounds have been marketed claiming to exert a controlling influence over bowel activity. However, most of these have an anticholinergic action and even Lomotil (diphenoxylate hydrochloride) contains 0.025 mgm. of atropine in each tablet.

Vegetable mucins are helpful when given in small repeated doses of half a teaspoonful (Isogel. Normacol, Metamucil, Celevac, etc.). They absorb water but care must be taken not to give larger doses or peristalsis will be stimulated.

Antibiotics should not be prescribed indiscriminately and wherever possible should only be used to counter a known infection. In the cases of 'holiday diarrhoea', it is reasonable to sanction iodochlorhydroxyquinoline (Enterovioform) since this will deal with the simple cases safely without exposing the patient to the risk of developing resistance should a dangerous pathogen supervene. The antibiotic management of infective diarrhoea is dealt with in Chapter 12.

Diet

This is now thought to be of less importance but it is reasonable to avoid stimulating the gastro-colic reflex. A fluid diet for 36 hours followed by small quantities of bland food at frequent intervals is a sensible régime.

Adequate fluids should always be given to compensate for the increased faecal loss. In cholera, fluid and electrolyte replacement is of extreme urgency.

CHAPTER 15

REGIONAL ENTERO-COLITIS (CROHN'S DISEASE)

Crohn's initial report in 1932 described fourteen cases of a non-specific granulomatous process involving the terminal ileum. Since that time far more widespread involvement of the alimentary tract has been recognised and different descriptive terms have been used i.e. terminal ileitis, regional enteritis, regional entero-colitis.

Recognition of the possibility of colonic involvement and distinction of these cases from classical ulcerative colitis is of considerable clinical significance, there being important differences in both prognosis and treatment between the two conditions.

Aetiology

The cause of the condition remains obscure.
 1 No specific bacterial agent has been isolated.
 2 Tuberculin skin tests are not more frequently positive than in controls.
 3 Specific food allergens have not been demonstrated.
 4 Auto-immunity is a possible but unproven factor.

Age and sex

The disease is most frequently encountered in young adults but may occur at any age. Sex incidence is approximately equal and geographical distribution is world-wide.

Pathology

The characteristic feature is a non-specific proliferative type of inflammatory reaction initially involving a limited length of

Regional Entero-colitis (Crohn's Disease)

the intestinal canal. Multiple segments may become affected, the intervening bowel appearing perfectly normal (skip lesions).

Any part of the gut from oesophagus to rectum may be involved but most commonly the condition occurs in the small intestine and in particular the terminal ileum. The colon may be involved in continuity with the ileum or the disease may be entirely confined to the large bowel.

1 Macroscopic features
   1 The mucosa and submucosa are predominantly involved but the muscle coat may be invaded and peritoneal reaction is common, the bowel appearing red and thickened.
   2 Mucosal ulceration occurs and gives a typical cobblestone appearance.
   3 The peritoneal reaction results in adhesions between loops of gut which may become obstructed.
   4 Regional lymph nodes may be enlarged.
   5 Fistula formation is common and may develop between contiguous loops of gut or appear externally in the perineum or through the abdominal wall. Deeper infiltration may subsequently cause abcess formation in the loin, buttock or elsewhere.

2 Microscopic features

If the following features are found then a definite diagnosis of Crohn's disease may be possible but in some cases the findings are not easy to interpret.
   1 Cellular infiltration with chronic inflammatory cells.
   2 Formation of epithelioid foci with giant cells.
   3 Marked oedema of the mucosa and submucosa.
   4 Hypertrophy of the muscle coat.
   5 Lymphatic obstruction and dilatation.

Clinical features

The most common presentation is that of a young adult with intermittent colicky abdominal pain and diarrhoea but cases may be first seen with more advanced disease with intestinal obstruction or abscess and fistula formation.

Symptoms:
1 Pain. This varies from mild colic and distension to severe pain associated with vomiting due to obstruction. Many cases present as acute appendicitis.
2 General health is often surprisingly well maintained except in the presence of extensive disease. Weight loss and general debility due to malabsorption and steatorrhoea are features of extensive small bowel involvement.
3 Diarrhoea is intermittent in most cases but may be a prominent feature in colonic involvement when the picture as a whole bears a close similarity to that of ulcerative colitis.
4 Fever is variable but occasionally it is persistent and Crohn's disease should be considered as a possibility when dealing with a pyrexia of unknown origin.
5 Frank bleeding is inconstant, even in those cases in which the large bowel is extensively involved. On the other hand, the faecal occult blood test is usually positive. In the more severe cases anaemia may be considerable and is usually of a simple hypochromic type due to chronic blood loss. More rarely it is megaloblastic, due to interference with folic acid or B_{12} absorption or due to the formation of a stagnant loop.

Signs:
1 There may be localised bowel tenderness or thickening and at times a palpable mass but examination is often negative in small bowel disease.
2 Fistula formation occurs sufficiently frequently to be considered as an integral part of the clinical picture rather than as a complication and occasionally it may be the presenting feature. The peri-anal area is the most frequently affected.
3 Large fleshy bluish coloured piles should suggest a diagnosis of Crohn's disease.

Investigations
1 Barium follow through will show areas of small bowel involvement. Narrowing of the terminal ileum (the string sign) and internal fistulae can be demonstrated.

Regional Entero-colitis (Crohn's Disease)

2 Barium enema will show colonic involvement but if the disease is confined to the colon, differentiation from idiopathic ulcerative colitis may be difficult.
3 Blood picture. There may be mild anaemia and leucocytosis and slight elevation of the sedimentation rate.
4 Rectal biopsy. This may be diagnostic but even when the rectum is involved the changes may be too nonspecific to make a diagnosis.
5 Laparotomy. This may be necessary to exclude other diseases and make a presumptive diagnosis of Crohn's. Surgical biopsy carries a risk of fistula formation. Enlarged mesenteric lymph nodes can be removed with safety.

Treatment

The principles of treatment in the majority of cases are conservative management for as long as possible with surgical intervention for complications where needed. This approach is taken because as yet there is no specific drug therapy for this disorder which is liable to recur even after resection.

Medical management:

Acute cases.
Bed rest and continuous gastric aspiration together with intravenous fluids and steroids result in the relief of a large number of subacute and acute obstructed cases. Many then go on to a complete clinical remission although the underlying disease remains.

Chronic cases.
Long term management is always a difficult problem but a careful diet and simple symptomatic measures backed by judicious use of steroids will enable the great majority of patients to enjoy a full life often for many years.

1 Diet
This should be as nutritious as possible so as to overcome loss from exudation and malabsorption. Indigestible residue should be avoided as this may precipitate obstruction.

2 Supplements
Haematinic therapy with iron, folic acid and vitamin B_{12} is

needed in severe cases. Additional potassium should be given to those with continuous diarrhoea.

3 Rest

Overfatigue should be avoided but normal activity encouraged. Periods of bed rest can be valuable in curtailing or preventing an incipient relapse. Sedatives sometimes alleviate colic better than analgesics.

4 Antispasmodics

A therapeutic trial of anticholinergic drugs is always indicated and often effective.

5 Antibacterial agents

Sulphonamides alone or in combination as Salazopyrin do not affect the disease process but may be helpful in cases where there is intestinal stasis or toxaemia from bacterial absorption. Broad spectrum antibiotics may be required in secondary abscess formation.

6 Oral steroids

These remain the standby although their action is purely non-specific. They can be used in either
  (i) Repeated courses, commencing as early as possible in any individual relapse with initial doses of 30—40 mgm. prednisone, progressively reducing as symptoms come under control
  or
  (ii) As long-term maintenance treatment, in which case a dose of 10 mg. of prednisone daily should be regarded as the maximum maintenance level.

Steroid enemas or suppositories may be helpful in distal colonic disease.

Surgical management

Surgery may be needed
  1 For the drainage of localised abscesses in the abdomen or perineum;

2 For the removal of fistulae;
3 For the treatment of obstructive episodes;
4 For the resection of affected gut in selected cases but aiming always to conserve as much effective bowel as possible.

CHAPTER 16

THE COLON AND RECTUM

Classification of disorders:
1. **Infections**
    - **(a) Bacillary dysentery**
    - **(b) Amoebic dysentery**
2. **Appendicitis**
3. **Disorders of structure and function**
    - **(a) Diverticular disease**
    - **(b) Irritable colon syndrome**
    - **(c) Hirschsprung's disease**
4. **Non-specific inflammatory disease**
    - **(a) Ulcerative colitis**
    - **(b) Regional enteritis**
5. **Tumours**
    - **(a) Malignant**
        - **(i) carcinoma**
        - **(ii) multiple familial polyposis**
        - **(iii) other tumours**
    - **(b) Benign**
        - **(i) adenomatous polyps**
        - **(ii) villous papilloma**
        - **(iii) other tumours**
6. **Vascular disorders**
    - **(a) Haemorrhoids**
    - **(b) Ischaemic colitis**

1 INFECTIONS

(a) Bacillary dysentery
(b) Amoebic dysentery

(see Chapter 12)

The Colon and Rectum 149

2 APPENDICITIS

Aetiology
1 Appendicitis most frequently results from obstruction of its lumen due to faecoliths or residues contained in food.
2 Rarely it occurs due to inflammation spreading directly from other local structures.

Pathology
There is stasis in the appendix with bacterial invasion of the wall and an inflammatory cellular reaction follows.

Because the appendix possesses a vulnerable vascular supply, gangrene as a result of thrombosis occurs early.

Clinical features
1 Pain is colicky and referred to the centre of the abdomen in the early stages. Localisation to the appendix area occurs when the parietal peritoneum becomes inflamed and is relatively late in the course of the disease. If the appendix is retrocaecal it may be absent.
2 Fever and tachycardia
3 Nausea and vomiting may occur with the pain.
4 There is usually a change in bowel habit, most commonly constipation but occasionally diarrhoea.
5 There is tenderness to pressure in the right iliac fossa and perhaps rebound tenderness in the left iliac fossa.
6 Rectal examination may reveal tenderness high on the right.

Investigations
There is usually a polymorphonuclear leucocytosis.

Treatment
This is surgical in the majority of cases and should be undertaken early to prevent general peritonitis occurring from rupture of a gangrenous appendix.

Differential diagnosis
Appendicitis may mimic many other acute intra-abdominal

disorders and the following must be considered:
1. Other gastroenterological causes of pain
   (i) Acute or perforated peptic ulcer
   (ii) Acute cholecystitis
   (iii) Gastro-enteritis
   (iv) Mesenteric adenitis, particularly in children and adolescents.
   (v) Crohn's disease (regional entero-colitis)
   (vi) Diverticulitis
   (vii) Acute intestinal obstruction.
2. Renal tract disease particularly pyelonephritis with renal colic.
3. Gynaecological disorders particularly salpingitis and tubal pregnancy.
4. Less commonly
   (i) basal chest infections with pleurisy
   (ii) herpes zoster
   (iii) the possibility of a carinoid tumour or carcinoma of the caecum as precipitating factors should also be borne in mind.

3 DISORDERS OF STRUCTURE AND FUNCTION

(a) Diverticular disease

Diverticula may occur in any part of the large bowel but the descending and sigmoid colon are the commonest sites. They are found with increasing frequency over the age of fifty and are more common in the obese. The saccules consist of mucosa and submucosa together with a thin layer of longitudinal muscle. They herniate through defects in the circular muscle between the taenia coli.

Pathology

In the majority of cases diverticula give rise to no symptoms but they are sites of potential infection. When inflammatory changes occur they are usually lowgrade and accompanied by an extensive pericolic reaction and abscesses may form in or just

The Colon and Rectum

outside the bowel wall. In some instances inflammation may be acute and occasionally early perforation occurs.

The bowel wall becomes oedematous and the muscular coat thickened. Narrowing of the lumen leads to partial obstruction. Later fibrosis dominates the picture and increases the obstruction.

Clinical features

The symptoms and signs largely depend on the extent of the inflammatory reaction associated with the diverticula.

Symptoms
1. Systemic reaction with fever and tachycardia
2. Abdominal pain may vary from a discomfort in the left iliac fossa to severe colicky pain.
3. Vomiting may occur with pain or with intestinal obstruction.
4. A change in bowel habit is common with constipation and/or diarrhoea.
5. Frank bleeding is less common than in ulcerative colitis but can be severe.

Signs
1. There may be localised tenderness over the inflamed area.
2. The affected length of bowel may be felt as a cylindrical thickening and a tender mass suggests abscess formation.

Investigations

1. Barium enema X-rays will demonstrate the extent of the diverticulosis and the degree of associated stenosis and spasm.

   Note:

   It may be difficult to differentiate between a localised area of diverticulitis and carcinoma or Crohn's disease. Either can occur in association with diverticular disease.
2. Sigmoidoscopy should be done to exclude a low carcinoma. In cases of diverticulitis the rectal mucosa is usually normal but may be slightly hyperaemic.
3. There is often a moderate polymorphonuclear leucocytosis and elevation of the sedimentation rate.

Treatment

Management should be aimed at:
1 Relieving pain and spasm with antispasmodics.
2 Preventing constipation and possible obstruction as far as possible by
   (a) advising a diet free of indigestible vegetable residue i.e. stalks, skins etc.
   (b) giving small quantities of hydrophilic agents (Isogel Celevac, Metamucil, Normacol) and also paraffin emulsion.
3 During the active stages and where a pericolic mass or even an abscess has formed, the initial treatment is still conservative. Bed rest and a fluid diet are indicated in the initial stages but later the traditional low residue diet may be permitted. Systemic antibiotics are appropriate and should be continued for some weeks since the inflammatory area is often densely walled.

Subsequently surgery may be necessary due to the persistence of sub-acute obstructive symptoms, drainage of an abscess or treatment of fistulae.

(b) Irritable colon syndrome

Other synonyms are: spastic colon, nervous colitis, mucus colitis and dyskinesia of the colon.

There is no doubt that many patients do experience considerable and long-continued discomfort clearly related to the colon, in whom no recognised disease process can be demonstrated. The patients are more commonly women than men and there is almost always a background of tension due to endogenous or environmental problems. The symptoms result from disordered bowel activity and mucus hypersecretion is frequently found.

Clinical features

Symptoms:
1 Recurrent attacks of abdominal discomfort or pain are the most common presentation. Pain may be in the left iliac fossa over the sigmoid, over the splenic and hepatic flexures or over the caecum. It is sometimes surprisingly severe and may simulate an acute abdomen.

The Colon and Rectum

2. Patients frequently complain of a lot of wind and may be relieved by passing it per rectum.
3. Constipation or diarrhoea may occur. The latter usually consists of the frequent passage of small amounts of faeces.
4. Weight loss is uncommon.
5. Anxiety and tension may be apparent.
6. The stools frequently contain an excess amount of mucus but blood is never seen.

Investigations

A Barium enema may show increased spasm during screening but apart from this investigations will be normal.

Diagnosis and treatment

1. These patients present a similar problem in management to those with nervous dyspepsia. The diagnosis should be made as far as possible on history and examination and the need for further investigations to exclude organic disease then considered i.e. blood count, stool examination, sigmoidoscopy and Barium enema.
2. Sympathetic explanation of the cause of the symptoms is essential.
3. Mild sedation with barbiturates i.e. Amylobarbitone 30—50 mgms. t.d.s. may be needed and in some cases psychiatric help should be sought.
4. Antispasmodics should be tried but rarely give complete relief.

(c) Hirschsprung's disease

In this disorder a segment of bowel fails to relax and contract normally due to a lack of myenteric ganglion cells. In the affected segment tone is persistently increased and this causes obstruction resulting in dilatation and hypertrophy of the colon proximal to it. The segment is usually in the rectum or sigmoid but may involve most of the colon. Boys are more frequently affected than girls.

Clinical features

The majority of cases present either
1. In infancy with abdominal obstruction and vomiting
   or
2. In childhood with failure to grow associated with constipation and distension.
3. A few cases reach adolescence before detection.

Investigations

1. Plain X-ray of the abdomen will show the gross colonic dilatation.
2. A Barium enema will confirm the colonic dilatation and careful examination may demonstrate a narrow segment.
3. A deep rectal biopsy, usually taken under anaesthesia, will show lack of ganglion cells in the nerve plexus.

Treatment

A colostomy will relieve the obstructive symptoms and constipation. When the bowel has been cleared, resection of the affected area and restoration of normal continuity can be carried out.

4 NON-SPECIFIC INFLAMMATORY DISEASE

(a) Ulcerative colitis (see Chapter 17)
(b) Regional entero-colitis (see Chapter 15)

5 TUMOURS

(a) Malignant

(i) Carcinoma

Sex: Colonic cancer has a slightly higher incidence in women whereas rectal cancer has a higher incidence amongst men.

Age: Both show an increasing incidence with age and are most common over the age of fifty.

Site: The majority of growths occur in the distal colon and more than half of these in the rectum itself.

The Colon and Rectum

Pathology

These tumours are epithelial in origin and arise from the columnar mucosa. Macroscopically they can be infiltrating, ulcerating or polypoid.

Microscopically they are scirrhous, adenomatous or colloid in type.

Clinical features

1. Rectal bleeding. Under no circumstances should rectal bleeding be ascribed to the presence of haemorrhoids without full examination to exclude the presence of a malignant lesion higher up.
2. Change in bowel habit (diarrhoea or constipation). The more proximal the lesion, the less definite is the clinical picture but any alteration of the bowel habit in the older patient should arouse suspicion.
3. Anaemia. Caecal and ascending colon growths are often symptomless but a proportion will still be detected in time if this diagnosis is remembered as a possibility in all cases of anaemia.
4. Sub-acute obstruction. This may occur with stenosing lesions.
5. Pain is a late feature and usually indicates advanced disease.

Investigations

1. Distal lesions can sometimes be seen sigmoidoscopically and confirmed by biopsy.
2. Barium enema. More proximal lesions are usually revealed by careful contrast radiography but tumours in the main body of the colon can escape detection.
3. The continued presence of blood, especially when confirmed sigmoidoscopically as coming from above the haemorrhoidal ring, should dictate a renewed search and exploratory laparotomy may be justified.

Treatment

If diagnosis is made early enough surgical resection gives good results. Present statistics show an average eight year survival rate of over 50% and this could be improved considerably if more careful note was taken of early signs.

Surgery is undertaken after preliminary preparation of the bowel by means of thorough lavage and the administration of a non-abscorbic antibiotic.

Aims of Treatment:
1. In early cases
    (a) Resection with restoration of continuity.
    (b) Removal of regional lymphatics.
2. In low rectal or advanced growths
    Abdomino-perineal excision may be necessary with the establishment of a permanent colostomy.
3. In cases with systemic secondaries
    Palliative relief of obstruction may be worthwhile.

(ii) Multiple Familial Polyposis

This should be considered premalignant (see Chapter 18).

(iii) Other Tumours

Carcinoid tumours arise from the argentaffin cells of the mucosa and squamous cell growths from the anal margin. A minority of growths (5% or so) are of mesenchymal origin and the commonest are of the lymphoma group. Other rarities include malignant melanoma and various types of sarcoma.

(b) Benign

(i) Adenomatous Polyps.
   These may occur singly or at several sites. The exact relationship of these to the development of carcinoma is uncertain but malignant change does occur in some.

(ii) Villous Papilloma.
   These rare tumours occur mainly in the distal colon and give rise to watery diarrhoea at times severe enough to produce collapse and dehydration due to fluid and electrolyte loss.

(iii) Other Tumours
   These include lipomas, angiomas and juvenile polyps.

The Colon and Rectum

6 VASCULAR DISORDERS

(a) Haemorrhoids

Haemorrhoids (piles) are distended rectal veins and since the rectum is one of the main sites of anastomosis between the portal and systemic venous systems their presence may signify more than local disease.

Aetiological factors

In the majority of cases there is no obvious cause but they may be due to
1. Intrapelvic mass causing obstruction
2. Portal hypertension
3. Local inflammatory disease i.e. Crohn's disease in which the haemorrhoids have a blue-purplish colour.

Pathology

Piles may bleed and cause anaemia and they may thrombose or prolapse.

Investigations

These should always include
   (a) Rectal examination
   (b) Proctoscopy
   (c) Sigmoidoscopy
   (d) Abdominal examination

to exclude other disease. If these suggest that there may be disease higher up, then a Barium enema may be necessary.

Treatment

Treatment is by astringent applications most conveniently in suppository form, sclerosing injections or surgical excision.

(b) Ischaemic colitis

(see Chapter 18)

CHAPTER 17
ULCERATIVE COLITIS

Definition

Ulcerative colitis consists of an inflammatory reaction of unknown cause involving the mucosa and submucosa of the large intestine.

Classification
1. **Distal colitis**
   (a) **Proctitis (rectum only)**
   (b) **Proctosigmoiditis (rectum and sigmoid)**
2. **Left-sided colitis (colon as far as splenic flexure)**
3. **Extensive colitis (colon to hepatic flexure)**
4. **Total colitis (whole colon)**
5. **Proximal colitis**
6. **Segmental colitis**

Note:
1. Cases of proctitis usually remain localised over many years.
2, 3 Proctosigmoiditis and left-sided colitis progress to more extensive disease in approximately 40% of cases.
4. In cases of total colitis there may be mild inflammatory changes in the distal few inches of the ileum but these are non-specific and resolve after colectomy.
5. Proximal colitis
   In rare cases the rectum may be radiologically and sigmoidoscopically normal when the more proximal colon is obviously abnormal. In these patients rectal biopsy will usually disclose microscopical evidence of involvement.
6. Segmental colitis
   In some cases only segments of the colon may be involved

Ulcerative Colitis

and a distinction between ulcerative colitis and Crohn's disease is often difficult and controversial.

Aetiology

1 The incidence is gradually but steadily increasing.
2 Young adults are predominantly affected but the condition may occur at any age.
3 No specific causative organisms have been isolated.
4 No single allergic factor has been found although some patient's symptoms are improved by the exclusion of certain foodstuffs (i.e. milk products) from the diet.
5 Psychological factors may figure prominently in the disease but whether these are of primary aetiological significance, part of the disease process or secondary to the disabilities of the disease is uncertain.

Pathology

In the early stages there is a simple inflammatory response with oedema, hyperaemia and moderate leucocytic infiltration without actual ulceration. The condition may never progress beyond this stage.

More severe involvement causes necrosis of the mucosa and frank ulceration. In acute cases the ulceration may be extensive. In chronic cases the combined effects of regeneration and destruction of the mucosa may give rise to the characteristic pseudo-polyp formation.

Involvement of the muscle coats only occurs when there is invasion by secondary bacterial infection in fulminating cases. The muscle then fails and the colon dilates giving rise to the appearances of megacolon.

The narrow, shortened colon seen in chronic colitis is the result of muscular spasm and hypertrophy.

Fibrosis is rarely a feature and stricture formation should be considered malignant until proved otherwise.

Clinical features—General features

Over half of patients have an insidious onset of symptoms with:
  mild abdominal discomfort

mild diarrhoea
occasional blood in the faeces

These symptoms gradually become more definite with diarrhoea particularly in the morning and with frequent blood and pus per rectum.

Approximately one-third of patients present with an acute attack with: fever
   diarrhoea
   marked loss of blood
   general malaise

and if untreated tend to deteriorate over a period of days or weeks.

Approximately one-tenth of patients present as fulminating cases with: profuse diarrhoea
   severe fluid and blood loss
   prostration.

These patients require emergency treatment and a high proportion come to early surgery.

The extent of the disease varies greatly but does not necessarily correlate with the severity of symptoms. Cases with total involvement tend to have a more severe local and systemic reaction but some patients continue for long periods in good health with minimal symptoms.

Conversely those with localised disease can be seriously ill.

Specific features:

1 Local bowel symptoms
2 Systemic symptoms
3 Local complications
4 Systemic complications.

Local bowel symptoms

(a) The passage of visible blood and mucus per rectum almost always occurs. These may be seen with the stool or may be passed without obvious faecal matter.
   Even in quiescent disease the stools will usually be positive for occult blood.

(b) Diarrhoea is not invariably a feature and it is important to find out whether this consists of fluid stools or only a

Ulcerative Colitis

frequent need to discharge small quantities of blood and mucus. In many cases of distal colitis, a normal if not constipated stool is passed between the frequent blood-stained discharges.
(c) Urgency of defaecation is characteristic of all types of ulcerative colitis and this with its attendant risk of incontinence, constitutes the patient's chief anxiety and incapacity. The demand for defaecation may occur one or twenty times a day and can prove exhausting and demoralising.
(d) Pain is not usually a presenting symptom although patients may have abdominal soreness and colic. Anal excoriation can cause distress.

Systemic symptoms

These are: weight loss
general debility
fever
and are associated with: tachycardia
dehydration
anaemia.

This systemic reaction is due to
1. Loss of water, electrolytes (Na., K., Mg.), blood and protein from the colonic wall into the faeces
2. Toxaemia and bacteraemia resulting from spread of colonic bacteria into the gut wall and subsequently into the portal and systemic circulation.

Local complications

These are: fissures and fistulae
haemorrhage
dilatation of the colon
perforation
carcinoma

Fissure may occur as a result of the diarrhoea and can be very distressing.

Fistulae are uncommon and when found should always raise the suspicion that the case is really an example of regional enterocolitis (Crohn's disease).

Severe haemorrhage occasionally occurs and may require emergency surgery.

Dilatation of the colon is a serious complication. It portends disintegration of the colon and is an indication for immediate colectomy in order to prevent multiple perforation. Disappearance of the diarrhoea in a severe colitic is an ominous sign and when accompanied by abdominal distension is virtually diagnostic of toxic megacolon, even though deterioration of the general condition may not immediately be apparent.

Perforation is rare except as a sequel to the colonic dilatation described above.

The risk of malignant change occurring increases with the extent and duration of the colitis; in total colitis the percentage incidence approximates to the duration of the disease in years i.e. a 20 year case will have a 20% risk of developing cancer, a 25 year case a 25% risk, etc. In cases involving the rectum only the risk of malignant change occurring is hardly above that of the normal population.

Systemic complications

1 Liver—fatty infiltration, pericholangitis, cirrhosis. These changes occur as a result of infection ascending via the portal system.
2 Eyes—iridocyclitis.
3 Joints—arthritis, sacro-iliitis, ankylosing spondylitis.
4 Skin—dermatitis, erythema, nodosum, pyoderma gangrenosum.

These groups of disorders are more frequently seen in the patients with active and extensive disease and their nature suggests an allergic or auto-immune mechanism.

5 Nervous system—psychological disturbances.

The psychological disturbances constitute a controversial subject. Some degree of mood change is almost invariable and frequently it is of severe degree. Colitic patients are notoriously difficult to manage, often have an irritatingly petulant attitude and being self-centred, disgruntled and ungrateful. They frequently exhibit immature traits and are peculiarly resistant to encouragement. The onset of the condition is commonly ascribed to anxiety situations.

The existence of these manifestations is not in dispute, the argument is as to whether they are an expression of inherent

Ulcerative Colitis

personality defects, predisposing to the development of the condition, or whether they are purely secondary manifestations due to the physical state. In support of the second viewpoint is the almost immediate restoration of mental balance following colectomy and this occurs in spite of the fact that the patient has a permanent ileostomy.

Investigations

1. Sigmoidoscopy. In mild cases there will be loss of the normal vascular pattern, a granular mucosa and a tendency for the mucosa to bleed on touch. In more severe cases there will be pus and blood in the rectum with a reddened ulcerated mucosa.
2. A plain X-ray of the abdomen is advisable in all cases of suspected colitis on admission. It may show:
    (i) dilatation of the colon
    (ii) faecal stasis proximal to distal disease.
3. Ba. enema X-rays will show the extent and severity of the disease. Points to look for are:
    (i) lack of definition of the mucosal outline
    (ii) lack of haustration
    (iii) ulceration and pseudo-polyp formation.
4. Rectal biopsy. Suction biopsy of the rectum provides the most satisfactory specimens for histology. In many cases the inflammatory changes are non-specific and it may be difficult to make a distinction from Crohn's disease.
5. Haematological examination may show anaemia and leucocytosis.
6. Serum chemistry may show electrolyte disturbances and evidence of protein loss.

Medical management

1. Sympathy and firm encouragement
2. Maintenance of restful but profitable activity
3. High quality diet
4. Control of bowel hyperactivity
5. Replacement medication
6. Antibacterial therapy

7 Steroid therapy
8 Continued surveillance

1 Sympathy and encouragement

It has to be emphasised that sympathetic understanding alone can result in considerable improvement in symptoms apart from giving comfort and therefore reducing the amount of sedation required.

2 Activity

The patient should be encouraged to remain at work as far as possible but undue fatigue should be avoided. In severe cases strict bed rest is essential.

3 Diet

The traditional low residue diet is unnecessarily restrictive and all too often is totally inadequate in keeping pace with the continuous drain of vital substances. So long as frank roughage is avoided, these patients should receive a full and even an above average diet.

4 Control of bowel hyperactivity

In colitis a great proportion of the fluid in the faeces is the result of serous exudation and for this reason complete control of diarrhoea is difficult. This point is of importance in cases of distal disease as severe stasis in the normal proximal bowel may result from over-treatment.

Anticholinergics are of value in some cases.

Codeine phosphate 30 mgms.—60 mgms. up to three or four times daily will frequently give considerable relief.

The regular use of opiates is contra-indicated in such a chronic disorder because of the possibility of addiction.

5 Replacement medication

Many cases of colitis are anaemic and will require intermittent if not continuous oral iron. A single daily tablet of ferrous sulphate (200 mgms.) is sometimes preferable to more liberal doses which result in default.

Ulcerative Colitis

Transfusion may be necessary in severe cases.

Potassium supplements may be needed if the disease is extensive.

6 *Antibacterial therapy*

Salicylazosulphapyridine (Salazopyrin) is both an antibacterial and anti-inflammatory agent and is used in dosages of up to 4 gms. daily to prevent relapses in patients who are in remission. It is of little value in acute relapse.

Systemic antibiotics may be needed in patients with toxaemia.

7 *Steroid therapy*

(a) Steroid suppositories are useful in the treatment of distal disease.
(b) Steroid retention enemas are self-administered and can be used alone or in conjunction with oral steroid therapy.
(c) Oral steroids are most effective in acute exacerbations. Long term administration is avoided where possible.
(d) Intramuscular A.C.T.H. is sometimes more effective than oral steroids in severe cases.

8 *Continued surveillance*

It is important to keep these patients under review
   (a) to try and anticipate acute exacerbations
   (b) to watch for complications and treat them early
   (c) to assess the risks of malignant change in long term cases.

Whilst early operation is obviously undesirable, the greatest possible care must be taken not to invoke the aid of the surgeon too late.

Surgical management

Surgery must be considered:
1. Where there are acute complications, i.e. toxic megacolon; perforation; severe haemorrhage.
2. Where medical treatment has failed in acute exacerbations of the disease.
3. Where there is chronic ill-health from colitis and the patient is unable to lead a reasonable life.

4 Where malignant change is suspected.
5 In long term cases with extensive disease who run a high risk of developing carcinoma.

The operations that may be performed are either:

1 Total colectomy

   When this operation is undertaken the disease cannot recur and the risk of malignancy is eliminated. However the patient has to accept the establishment of a permanent ileostomy

or

2 Subtotal colectomy and ileo-rectal anastomosis

   This procedure has a higher primary morbidity and mortality and in addition the risk of rectal cancer remains.

Choice between the two methods is very much an individual matter and although many surgeons consider the former to be the method of choice, the latter procedure should be given serious consideration especially in young patients who have short histories.

CHAPTER 18

RARER GASTRO-INTESTINAL CONDITIONS

The following are discussed in this chapter:
> **Ectopic gastric mucosa**
> **Pancreatic heterotopia**
> **Zollinger-Ellison syndrome**
> **Carcinoid tumours**
> **Peutz-Jeghers syndrome**
> **Multiple familial polyposis**
> **Chronic ischaemic colitis**
> **Pneumatosis cystoides intestinalis**
> **Whipple's disease**
> **Progressive systemic sclerosis**

ECTOPIC GASTRIC MUCOSA

Aetiology
Actively secreting gastric mucosa is:
1 Always found in Meckel's diverticulum
2 At times found in the oesophagus
   (a) rarely as isolated mucosal islands at any point along its length
   (b) more frequently lining the phrenic ampulla and lower oesophagus in direct continuity with the gastric lining.

Pathology
Both regions are potential sites for the development of peptic ulceration and its complications of haemorrhage, perforation and fibrosis.

Clinical features
1 Meckel's diverticulum
   Patients may present with the symptoms of recurring abdominal pain after food referred to the centre or lower abdomen. A clinical diagnosis is often difficult and the diverticulum may only be shown on a Barium follow-through or discovered at laparotomy.
2 Oesophagus
   Ectopic mucosa in this site presents a clinical picture very similar to that produced by oesophageal reflux with heartburn and pain on swallowing.

PANCREATIC HETEROTOPIA

Aetiology

Although a comparative rarity, this disorder was recognised over 200 years ago. It is seldom diagnosed clinically, the true nature of the lesion only being discovered on histological examination of resected specimens.

Pathology

The ectopic lesion most commonly takes the form of a small marble-sized nodule in the wall of the pyloric antrum or duodenum. Half the deposits are within 5 cm. of either side of the pylorus but a few are found in the biliary system or small intestine.

The nodule may consist of any or all of the components of pancreatic tissue including islet cells and can be affected by any of the disorders that occur in a normally placed pancreas.

Clinical features

The symptoms are similar to those of a chronic duodenal or pyloric canal ulcer but if the nodule is in the small intestine, it may present with intussusception.

Treatment
1 Simple enucleation is possible if the condition is recognised preoperatively.

2 Extensive resection is not advocated but is often carried out as the lesion is so often mistaken for an ulcer or a carcinoma.

THE ZOLLINGER-ELLISON SYNDROME

Aetiology

In spite of the rarity of this syndrome it is remarkable that it eluded recognition until late 1955 for the clinical features are striking. The syndrome is due to islet cell tumours of the pancreas which produce gastrin causing excessive gastric secretion.

Pathology

The tumours vary in size from 2—10 mm. in diameter and may be found anywhere in the pancreas. About one-fifth are outside the pancreas. Half are reported as being malignant and metastases are usually present.

Occasionally no actual tumour is present and in these cases a diffuse adenomatosis of the islet cells will be found.

Clinical features

1 Intractable peptic ulceration is usual, multiple lesions often being present which sometimes extend well down into the jejunum.
2 Haemorrhage or perforation is frequent.
3 Persistent diarrhoea may be present due to
    (a) irritation of the small intestine by the acid
    (b) simple failure to absorb the excess gastric secretion
    (c) inactivation of pancreatic enzymes by the lowered pH. This also results in steatorrhoea.

Investigations

1 Gastric function tests
    These show a voluminous gastric secretion with an equally high acid content. Overnight secretion may be well in excess of two litres with an HCl output of over 100

mEq/litre. (Normal findings are less than half a litre with a total acid content of only 15—20 mEq.).
2 Barium meal and follow-through X-ray may show
   (a) gastric, duodenal or jejunal ulceration
   (b) rapid transit through the small intestine and an abnormal mucosal pattern.

Treatment
1 Even in those cases in which a definite pancreatic tumour is located and excised, treatment is disappointing.
2 Extensive or total gastric resection may be needed to alleviate symptoms.
3 Vagotomy is of no value as the hypersecretion is due to hormonal and not vagal stimulation.

CARCINOID TUMOURS

Aetiology
Kultschitzky at the end of the last century was the first to observe the presence of chromaffin cells in the intestinal mucosa and these continue to bear his name. It was later found that they contained silver reducing cytoplasmic granules and this earned them a new title of argentaffin cells. They secrete serotonin (5 hydroxytryptamine), which has a stimulatory effect upon smooth muscle.

Pathology
Tumours arising from these specialised cells are known as carcinoids or argentaffinomas. The gastrointestinal tract, the blood vessels and the bronchi may all be involved.

The main sites for these tumours are the appendix and the terminal ileum. A small benign nodule is frequently found on routine histology in appendicectomy specimens. Larger tumours are fortunately rare, since most of them are malignant.

Clinical features
These consist of increased intestinal activity (borborygmi and diarrhoea), facial flushing, syncopal episodes and bronchospasm. These effects are due to excess of circulating serotonin.

Investigations

The urinary excretion of 5 hydroxyindole acetic acid (5 H.I.A.A.) will be increased above the normal of 3—8 mgms./24 hours.

Treatment

Treatment consists of surgical removal. Even in the malignant cases the prognosis for survival is surprisingly good, especially if the secondary deposits can also be removed.

PEUTZ-JEGHERS SYNDROME

Aetiology

The syndrome is characterised by numerous adenomatous polyps of the intestine and pigmentation of the lips and mouth. The condition is familial and is probably transmitted by a Mendelian dominant gene. There is no particular sex or race predominance and the most usual time of presentation is in adolescence.

Pathology

1 Pigmentation
   The macules tend to be round or oval and brownish in colour. There is an increased number of melanin cells deep in the epithelium and melanophores in the underlying fibrous tissue.
2 Polyps
   These are usually multiple and vary in size from the microscopic to being large enough to cause obstruction. They may occur from the mouth to the rectum but are most common in the small intestine. Histologically the stroma contains smooth muscle and may show marked branching. The mucosal elements are normal in structure and proportions. Although active mitosis can be found, malignant change is uncommon.

Clinical features

1 The disorder may be diagnosed at sight because of the skin pigmentation. On the face these melanin deposits are usually at first mistaken for freckles but closer observa-

tion will reveal that they cross the muco-cutaneous boundaries and are numerous on the lips and within the mouth. They may also be observed on the trunk and limbs.
2 Obstruction due to intussusception is a common mode of presentation. A preceding history of intermittent and unexplained colic is often obtained.
3 Melaena is not uncommon.
4 The stomach may also be involved and on rare occasions polyps have appeared in the vomit.
5 There may be other associated abnormalities such as finger clubbing or ovarian tumours.

Investigations

1 A Barium meal and follow-through or a Barium enema may demonstrate polyps.
2 Gastroscopy and sigmoidoscopy may demonstrate the lesions if the stomach or rectum is involved.
3 The stools are often positive for occult blood.

Treatment

Surgery is indicated for the removal of polyps causing complications. Total clearance of polyps from the bowel is usually impracticable and new lesions may be expected to appear later. The vast majority of cases are benign.

MULTIPLE FAMILIAL POLYPOSIS (POLYPOSIS COLI)

Aetiology

This is a familial disease, fortunately rare, but half the progeny of an affected individual may also expect to have the condition.

Pathology

These adenomatous polyps develop *only* in the colon and are multiple. They are potentially very highly malignant.

Clinical features

These are variable and do not usually appear until early adult life. Irregular bowel activity with occasional bleeding is the usual picture but severe anaemia may be the first indication.

Investigations
1. Sigmoidoscopy will demonstrate the polyps as the rectum is always involved.
2. A Barium enema will show the extent and degree of colonic involvement.

Treatment
Colectomy is essential because of the high risk of malignancy. While total colectomy removes this risk, ileo-rectal anastomosis may be justified provided there is careful follow-up. A thorough sigmoidoscopy should be performed at six-monthly intervals so that any new polyps can be either fulgurated or excised.

ISCHAEMIC COLITIS

Aetiology
The mid-section of the colon (mid-transverse to mid-descending) is supplied by a marginal artery which is an anastomotic link between the superior and inferior arteries. Such an arrangement makes it more likely that damage will result to the bowel from an occlusive or hypotensive episode. Such episodes are more likely in elderly patients.

Pathology
1. Transient ischaemia may be followed by complete healing.
2. More severe ischaemia may fall short of total destruction of the gut wall but will be followed by fibrous repair and stricture formation.
3. Ischaemia may be severe enough to cause necrosis of the gut wall which leads to peritonitis due to bacterial invasion.

Clinical features
Patients may present
1. with subacute obstruction due to stricture formation
2. as an emergency with sudden diarrhoea and rectal bleeding with signs of peritonitis.

Investigations

1 A Barium enema may be possible in subacute and chronic cases and will demonstrate local strictures or tubular narrowing.
2 Aortography may be helpful in selected patients but in the age group involved is likely to show extensive vascular defects.

Treatment

1 Laparotomy and resection in acute severe cases.
2 Resection of local strictures in cases of obstruction.

PNEUMATOSIS CYSTOIDES INTESTINALIS

Aetiology

This condition consists of multiple gas-filled cysts situated within the wall of the bowel (either subserosally or submucosally). The jejunum is the commonest site but both ileum and colon can be involved, as can the mesentery, the peritoneum and even the lymph nodes. The origin of the air is unknown but a large percentage of cases also have asthma, pulmonary disease or an upper gastro-intestinal lesion such as a peptic ulcer.

Clinical features

1 It is probable that most cases are entirely asymptomatic
2 There may be mild diarrhoea and traces of blood per rectum
3 Occasionally the cysts may rupture intra-peritoneally, or one may be large enough to give rise to intussusception.

Investigations

1 Sigmoidoscopy may show the cysts if the rectum is involved. The cysts usually have the appearance of smooth, rounded sessile polyps.
2 Plain X-rays of the abdomen and Barium studies will confirm the diagnosis and extent of the disease.

Rarer Gastro-intestinal Conditions 175

Treatment

There is no known medical means of treating these cysts and surgical intervention is rarely required.

WHIPPLE'S DISEASE

Aetiology

This is a systemic disease most commonly occurring in males. The aetiology is unknown but bacilliform bodies have been demonstrated on electronmicroscopy in the submucosa and enterococci have been isolated from this area. Whether these are the organisms responsible for the disease is not certain but the disorder does respond to antibiotics.

Pathology

There is heavy infiltration of the submucosa of the intestine with large macrophages containing a glycoprotein which can be well demonstrated with the per-iodic acid Schiff stain. Although the epithelium appears normal, the villi become thickened and blunted. The infiltration causes lymphatic obstruction and steatorrhoea. Similar macrophages may be found in mesenteric and other lymph nodes.

Clinical features

Cases may present
1. In subacute form with fever, loss of weight, diarrhoea, lymphadenopathy and arthropathy. Untreated these patients die in about six months.
2. In a more chronic form with less severe malabsorption.
3. With arthropathy, which can precede other symptoms by several years.

Investigations

1. Xylose absorption tests and faecal fat estimation will confirm intestinal malabsorption and steatorrhoea.
2. A Barium follow-through X-ray will show a 'malabsorption pattern' with coarse mucosal folds.

3 Peroral small gut biopsy will show evidence of subepithelial infiltration with macrophages and confirm the diagnosis.
4 Rectal and lymph node biopsy may also demonstrate P.A.S. staining macrophages.

Treatment

1 Antibiotics such as Tetracycline or Chloramphenicol may keep patients in clinical remission.
2 Steroid therapy may be required in addition to antibiotics in order to obtain a remission.

PROGRESSIVE SYSTEMIC SCLEROSIS (SCLERODERMA)

Aetiology

This is a systemic disorder of connective tissue most commonly affecting adult females. Abnormalities of the immunoglobulins are frequently found but the exact aetiology is unknown.

Pathology

The disorder commonly affects the skin, joints, muscles, lungs and the intestine. The intestinal changes are principally those of atrophy of the submucosa together with progressive replacement of the smooth muscle by fibrous connective tissue which leads to impaired gut motility. As a result of this impairment, oesophageal reflux may occur, the lower oesophagus may become inflamed and strictures may develop.

Clinical features

1 Dysphagia and retrosternal discomfort due to oesophageal reflux can be distressing.
2 Intermittent ileus or steatorrhoea and malabsorption may result from small intestinal involvement.
3 Constipation can occur as a result of colonic involvement.
4 Skin changes almost always are present if there is intestinal disease.

Investigations

1. Barium swallow, follow-through and enema may demonstrate disordered function in any part of the gut.
2. Oesophageal manometry will confirm the abnormal oesophageal motility.
3. Oesophagoscopy and direct oesophageal biopsy may help confirm the diagnosis.
4. Absorption tests will be abnormal in cases of steatorrhoea.

Treatment

There is no specific remedy and symptomatic measures are required.

1. Small, easily swallowed and digested meals, together with antacids, will relieve dysphagia and dyspepsia.
2. Gentle laxatives may relieve constipation.
3. Steroids may temporarily alleviate the symptoms but have not been proved to have any significant effect on the course of the disease.
4. Antibiotics may occasionally be helpful in cases of malabsorption.

CHAPTER 19

INVESTIGATION TECHNIQUES

Although a full history and physical examination are of primary importance in the analysis of digestive disorders, a number of procedures are available to assist in the diagnosis.

While the existence of totally unsuspected disease may occasionally be disclosed as a result of these investigation techniques, their chief value lies in confirmation or assessment of a clinical diagnosis. Negative results must never be relied upon to exclude disease in the face of suggestive clinical findings.

The investigations more commonly used are discussed under the following headings
- **1 Examination of Vomit**
- **2 Examination of Faeces**
- **3 Endoscopy**
- **4 Radiography**
- **5 Radioactive Studies**
- **6 Mucosal Biopsy**
- **7 Motility Studies**
- **8 Specific Function Tests**
  - **(a) Gastric**
  - **(b) Hepatic**
  - **(c) Pancreatic**
  - **(d) Small intestinal**
- **9 Liver biopsy**

1 EXAMINATION OF VOMIT

The clinician must take the opportunity of examining the vomit himself wherever possible in all patients. Points to note are:
1 Volume of vomit (this may be very large in cases of pyloric obstruction).

Investigation Techniques

2 Appearance, colour and presence of undigested food.
3 Presence of frank or occult blood.

2 EXAMINATION OF FAECES

The clinician should not rely on reported macroscopic abnormalities but should examine the faecal specimens himself and this should be considered an essential part of the clinical examination.

1 Volume. In diarrhoeal states measurement of the volume of fluid lost in the faeces is essential in assessing the replacement requirement.
2 Appearance. The colour should be noted as it will vary in such disorders as jaundice and gastrointestinal haemorrhage and during oral drug treatment particularly with iron. In gross steatorrhoea the stools may be greasy. The presence of frank blood, mucus and parasites should be looked for.
3 Occult blood. Testing for the presence of occult blood is a simple and routine procedure. It can be carried out at the bedside with faeces obtained on rectal examination or in the laboratory on collected specimens. During the test the speed of appearance and intensity of colour change can be roughly quantitated with the amount of blood present in the sample.

Microscopy and Culture

For the examination of ova, cysts and parasites wet preparations should be made from fresh specimens of faeces. It is essential that a fresh, warm, semi-liquid stool is obtained when looking for amoebae.

The presence of fat globules or undigested meat fibres should be noted.

Aerobic and anaerobic cultures should be set up in the search for pathogenic bacteria. In cases of severe staphylococcal infection or moniliasis, a Gram film will also be helpful.

3 ENDOSCOPY

1 Oesophagoscopy

Indications:
(a) Removal of foreign bodies

(b) Diagnosis in cases of dysphagia
(c) Confirming the presence of oesophageal varices
(d) Examination and biopsy of areas considered suspicious on a Barium swallow.

Examination of the oesophagus can be carried out with rigid or with flexible fibre-optic instruments. Both give an adequate view but the latter cause less discomfort, reduce the risk of perforation and enable the procedure to be performed in elderly kyphotic patients in whom it would not otherwise be practicable.

2 Gastroscopy

Indications:

(a) In cases of acute haemorrhage where acute erosions are suspected.
(b) Where a gastric lesion is suspected and Barium meal shows no obvious abnormality.
(c) Confirmation of diagnosis in selected cases where X-rays have shown abnormality.

As with oesophagoscopy, the procedure should be considered complementary to radiology. Gastroscopy may be carried out with semi-rigid or with flexible fibre-optic instruments. The later have the advantages of allowing the stomach to be examined in the ward or out-patient clinic with very little disturbance of the patient.

A photographic record of lesions seen can be made by having a camera attached to or incorporated in the gastroscope. Many instruments now also allow for biopsies to be taken under direct vision.

Lesions high in the stomach may be difficult or impossible to see. Good views of the body and pyloric antrum can be expected but information of value is rarely obtained from the duodenal cap with the instruments at present available.

3 Peritoneoscopy

This procedure involves the creation of a pneumo-peritoneum and then the introduction of the peritoneoscope into the peritoneal cavity. It is extensively used on the continent of Europe but its use is limited in this country.

Investigation Techniques 181

Indications:
- (a) Examination of the liver and peritoneum for secondary deposits in cases of carcinoma so as to avoid unnecessary laparotomy.
- (b) The obtaining of liver biopsies under direct vision.
- (c) Examination of the upper abdominal viscera when the diagnosis may be in question.

4 Proctoscopy and Sigmoidoscopy

These procedures must always be preceded by digital rectal examination.

Indications:
- (a) Provided that there is no contra-indication these should be considered part of the examination in most cases of gastro-intestinal disorder and in all cases of diarrhoea, constipation or rectal bleeding.
- (b) For the follow-up assessment of distal inflammatory disease i.e. ulcerative colitis.
- (c) In follow-up of cases where polyps have been removed.

These procedures can be carried out on a firm couch in the left lateral position, the knee-elbow position or on a modification of the knee-elbow position on a tilting table. In the majority of cases prior preparation is not needed.

Rectal bipsies and mucosal swabs can be taken through either instrument.

4 RADIOGRAPHY

1 Plain Abdominal Film

In cases of suspected abdominal disorder the plain film can often prove to be equal in value to the chest film in chest diseases and should be undertaken more frequently as a screening procedure.

It is of particular value:
- (a) In cases of intestinal obstruction by demonstrating distended loops of bowel and fluid levels.
- (b) In cases of abdominal pain when the presence of gallstones, pancreatic calcification or renal stones may be noted.

(c) In the diagnosis of carcinoma of the stomach, ulcerative colitis with pseudo-polyposis and pneumatosis cystoides intestinalis spontaneous air contrast may occasionally be of help.
(d) In cases of ascending cholangitis air may be sometimes seen in the biliary tree.
(e) Hydatid cysts may be seen in liver or spleen.

2 Barium Contrast Studies

1 Barium swallow and meal
Indications:
  (a) Cases of dyspepsia that are persistent, recurrent or fail to respond to simple measures quickly.
  (b) All cases of dysphagia.
  (c) Suspected cases of hiatus hernia, oesophageal reflux, peptic ulceration or carcinoma.
  (d) In the differential diagnosis of retrosternal pain where there is doubt as to whether it is cardiac or gastro-intestinal in origin.
  (e) In the differential diagnosis of frank or occult bleeding from the upper gastro-intestinal tract.

2 Barium follow through
Indications:
  (a) Cases of malabsorption and steatorrhoea.
  (b) Cases of diarrhoea of undetermined origin.
  (c) Cases of suspected disaccharidase deficiency both with and without specific sugars by mouth.
  (d) In the differential diagnosis of frank or occult bleeding from the upper gastro-intestinal tract.

3 Barium enema
Indications:
  (a) Cases of rectal bleeding when the source is above the reach of the sigmoidoscope.
  (b) Where there has been an unexplained recent change in bowel habit.
  (c) Cases of diarrhoea unexplained after small intestinal studies.
  (d) When colonic disease is suspected because of pain of the presence of a mass, etc.

Investigation Techniques

(e) Assessment of the extent of colonic disease in ulcerative colitis and diverticulitis.

A large part of interpretation of these studies lies in direct observations made by the radiologist on screening. In this context it is important to remember that the value of the radiologist's opinion is directly proportional to the amount of information he receives from the clinician.

3 Biliary Tract

1 Oral cholecystography

Indications:
   (a) All cases of suspected gallbladder disease where jaundice is absent or slight.
   (b) In the differential diagnosis of atypical upper abdominal pain.
   (c) In the assessment of gallbladder function when gallstones are noted on a plain X-ray.

2 Intravenous cholangiography

Indications:
   (a) In cases where the common bile duct needs to be studied specifically.
   (b) In cases where oral cholecystography shows a non-functioning gallbladder. This technique may outline the biliary duct system.
   (c) Post-cholecystectomy complications.
   (d) In cases where oral cystography is not practicable i.e. because of vomiting.

In cases of obstructive jaundice the likelihood of obtaining worthwhile films with these techniques decreases with the intensity of the jaundice. Such cases however usually come to laparotomy and then the following surgical techniques may be considered:

   (i) Percutaneous transhepatic cholangiography may prove useful to the surgeon in determining the site of the obstruction but it should be considered as a pre-operative procedure owing to the risk of haemorrhage or bile peritonitis.
   (ii) Direct operative cholangiography is used in outlining the biliary tree in difficult cases and in ensuring that no stones remain in the common duct.

4 Angiography

1 Mesenteric and pancreatic arteries

Selective catheterisation of these arteries through a femoral puncture can be achieved and may be helpful in selected cases of ischaemic enteritis and pancreatic tumour. Experience with these techniques is limited to certain centres only at the present time.

2 Portal venography

It may be helpful to outline the portal venous system in suspected cases of portal vein obstruction or portal hypertension. Contrast medium can be injected percutaneously into the spleen, into the hepatic vein through a catheter passed down from a vein in the upper limb or directly into a branch of the portal vein at operation.

5 RADIOACTIVE STUDIES

1 Scanning

1 Liver

External scintillation counting over the liver area can be carried out after the injection of radioactive gold, iodinated albumin or iodinated Rose Bengal. It is particularly useful in determining the presence of space occupying lesions of the liver and if metastases are demonstrated in a case of cancer, unnecessary surgery may be avoided.

2 Pancreas

Similar scanning over the pancreas may identify tumours. Results are not as easy to interpret as with the liver.

2 Blood Loss

Examination of intestinal aspirate or faeces after an intravenous injection of radioactive iron or chromium tagged red cells may be helpful in the diagnosis of the site and degree of gastrointestinal bleeding.

Investigation Techniques

6 MUCOSAL BIOPSY

1 Gastric Biopsy

Samples of mucosa can be obtained without recourse to surgery both under direct vision through a gastro-scope or by means of suction biopsy capsule.

Indications:
- (a) The former method is of use in localised lesions such as carcinoma.
- (b) The latter method being 'blind' is only suitable for diffuse lesions such as the various types of gastritis.

2 Peroral Small Intestinal Biopsy

A number of suction biopsy instruments are available for taking mucosal samples. The instrument should be passed into the required position under X-ray screening control.

Indications:
- (a) In the differential diagnosis of steatorrhoea.
- (b) To confirm the diagnosis of diffuse disease of the small gut such as gluten enteropathy.
- (c) To follow the response of diffuse disease after treatment.

3 Rectal Biopsy

Such biopsies can be obtained through a proctoscope or sigmoidoscope either with biopsy forceps or with a suction biopsy instrument. Specimens obtained by suction biopsy are easier to interpret histologically as there is less trauma to the tissue. forceps biopsy is more practicable in local tumours.

Indications:
- (a) Diagnosis of inflammatory and infiltrative disease.
- (b) Diagnosis of malignancy.
- (c) Assessment of the possibility of pre-cancerous change in ulcerative colitis.

7 MOTILITY STUDIES

These are still mostly employed in the study of normal physiological function but are being increasingly used in abnormal states.

Pressure studies can be made with open-ended catheters or balloons in the oesophagus, stomach and colon. Motility studies can be made using free telemetering capsules ('radio-pills').

8 SPECIFIC FUNCTION TESTS

1 Gastric Function Tests

(a) The augmented histamine test, the histamine analogue 'histalog' (3 beta aminophthyl-pyrazole) test or stimulation with pentagastrin will demonstrate the capacity of the stomach for acid secretion. In patients with abdominal pain a high acid output may suggest a duodenal ulcer and achlorhydria will be found in cases of pernicious anaemia.

(b) The 'Diagnex' tubeless test for gastric acidity is a useful screening procedure in cases of anaemia.

2 Hepatic Function Tests

These tests are based upon the following:

(a) Bilirubin excretion
(b) Protein metabolism
(c) Carbohydrate metabolism
(d) Lipid metabolism
(e) Enzyme activity
(f) Dye excretion

(a) Bilirubin Excretion

The total serum bilirubin level gives a useful quantitative estimate of the intensity of jaundice but in cases of hepatitis is not necessarily proportional to the degree of hepatic damage.

The 'indirect' and 'direct' reactions (indicative respectively of free or conjugated bilirubin), help to differentiate between hepatocellular and obstructive jaundice by determining whether or not the bilirubin has passed through the liver cell. Although both are almost invariably raised in any case of jaundice the predominant reaction tends to be 'indirect' in the hepato-cellular and 'direct' in the obstructive type.

The total is usually less than 0.5 mgm.%, 0.3 mgm.% being free (indirect reaction) and 0.2 mgm.% conjugated (direct reaction).

The urinary pigments also give some guide as to the type of jaundice since only conjugated bilirubin (direct) can pass the renal filter and so give rise to bilirubinuria. Unconjugated bilirubin in haemolytic states may reach a very high level in the serum (15 mgm. or more) without appearing in the urine (acholuric jaundice).

Urobilinogen is formed by bacterial action in the intestine and therefore reabsorption and re-excretion of this type (urobilinogenuria) can only occur if the liver cells are still functioning i.e. in the early stages of hepato-cellular disease and pure haemolytic jaundice. The one exception is in the presence of infective cholangitis when the bacteria within the liver are able to form urobilinogen.

(b) Protein Metabolism

The liver plays an important part in the metabolism of proteins and in advanced insufficiency from any cause the serum albumen levels fall (normal: 3.5—5.0 gm.%).

Changes in the globulin fractions are a more sensitive indication of hepato-cellular dysfunction and these are the basis of the 'flocculation reactions'. The colloidal gold, the thymol turbidity, the zinc sulphate, the ammonium chloride, etc. are all responses to various globulin fractions.

Paper electrophoresis is a more refined method of fractionating the various serum proteins but otherwise is not of any additional advantage in the differential diagnosis of liver disease.

Hypoprothrombinaemia is usual in liver insufficiency states but is not specific to any particular type.

The blood ammonia level rises in the presence of liver damage and is probably one of the causes of the neurological manifestations in hepatic failure.

(c) Carbohydrate Metabolism

Since the liver cells are almost exclusively concerned with the conversion of galactose to glycogen, the galactose tolerance is a fairly critical indicator of hepatic cell function. Provided intestinal absorption is unimpaired this test, although infrequently used, remains one of the more reliable means of distinguishing between hepatocellular and obstructive jaundice.

(d) Lipid Metabolism

The serum cholesterol level provides a somewhat less critical distinction but values tend to be high in obstructive jaundice and low in hepato-cellular disease.

(e) Enzyme Tests

The serum alkaline phosphatase level is a sensitive indicator which is more markedly and consistently raised in obstructive than in hepato-cellular jaundice. It is also frequently elevated in hepatic carcinomatosis before jaundice is clinically apparent.

The serum transaminase levels are more suggestive of cellular dysfunction although again they may be raised when there are obstructive lesions. The glutamic pyruvic (S.G.P.T.) level invariably exceeds the glutamic oxalo-acetic (S.G.O.T.) in severe liver cell damage.

Lactic dehydrogenase (L.D.H.) has been incompletely evaluated as yet, but may prove useful as a differentiating measure when other causes for raised alkaline phosphatase co-exist, such as bone disease.

(f) Dye Excretion

Dyes serve as a means of detecting the presence of liver dysfunction in the absence of jaundice but are of no value in the differentiation between the types of jaundice.

Bromsulphthalein is readily taken up by the healthy liver and no more than 4% of the administered intravenous dose should still be retained in the circulation after 45 minutes. However, in the presence of hepatic disease this figure may rise to 20% or more.

Rose Bengal is handled similarly by the liver but its facility for combining with ^{131} enables external scanning techniques to be employed in addition to allowing calculations of uptake and rates of disappearance from the circulation to be made.

3 Pancreatic Function Tests

(a) The serum amylase and lipase levels may provide a guide

in the acute pancreatic disorders. In acute haemorrhagic pancreatitis the serum amylase levels may rise very high, at times over 1000 Somogyi units (normal 80—150) but it must be remembered that a single injection of morphia may result in considerable elevation of the level in the absence of any pancreatic disease, as a result of spasm of the sphincter of Oddi.

In less acute cases the serum enzyme levels which depend on the degree of duct obstruction and excretory capacity of the gland are less reliable.

(b) Secretin which stimulates the electrolyte and fluid production and pancreozymin which stimulates the exocrine enzyme production, can be used in the diagnosis of pancreatic insufficiency.

Duodenal aspirations and blood samples taken before and after intravenous injection of secretin and pancreozymin enable the volume, bicarbonate and enzyme output of the pancreas to be estimated. Worth-while information can only be obtained in experienced hands where the tests are performed regularly under standard conditions.

4 Small Intestinal Absorption Tests

1 Dietary Fat Absorption

This is the most consistent indicator of the absorptive capacity of the small bowel since it is almost invariably involved in all types of malabsorption defects. It is also a sensitive measure since the normal individual should assimilate at least 95% of the dietary fat intake and even a fall to 90% is indicative of a significant absorption defect.

The most reliable method of assaying fat absorption is the chemical analysis of a three or five day faecal collection. In practice it is not necessary to measure the daily fat intake but it is important to ensure that it is at least 75 gm. The average daily stool fat content should not exceed 5—7 gm.

Other techniques employ radio-isotope (131 I) labelled fats for subsequent tracing in either the blood or the stool. Unfortunately both false positive and false negative results may occur. Both neutral fat (triolein) and free fatty acid (oleic acid) have been used.

2 Carbohydrate Absorption

(a) Monosaccharides

The standard glucose tolerance test may help in differentiating between intestinal and pancreatic steatorrhoea. In intestinal steatorrhoea a relatively small rise in blood sugar of less than 40 mgms.% above the fasting level (flat curve) is usual after 50 gms. of oral glucose. Flat curves however may also occur in patients severely ill from any cause. In pancreatic insufficiency a high curve may be obtained due to islet cell damage resulting in insulin deficiency and impaired glucose metabolism.

D-xylose is widely employed and has two advantages for use in testing for intestinal absorptive function. It is (a) passively absorbed and (b) poorly metabolised so that blood and urine levels may be expected to be more specifically related to any intestinal defect. If renal function is normal, excretion of 20% or less of the ingested xylose suggests a mucosal absorptive defect.

(b) Disaccharides

The enzymes concerned in reducing the disaccharides to monosaccharides operate within the mucosal cell of the small intestine, thus highly specific deficiency syndromes can exist due to congenital absence of one or other of these enzymes (lactase—sucrase—maltase—invertase).

Their existence can be detected by the performance of the relevant suger tolerance test which is carried out in an exactly comparable way to the glucose tolerance test.

3 Protein Absorption

This is less consistently disturbed in malabsorption states although faecal nitrogen excretion above the normal average of 2.2—2.5 gm. (on a 100 gm. diet) has been recorded in 58% of cases of 'non-tropical sprue'. Figures tend to be higher in pancreatic insufficiency but are still inconsistent.

It is also possible to carry out more specific tests by directly assaying di-peptide absorption.

4 Haematinics

Iron and folic acid are normally mainly absorbed in the upper small intestine and vitamin B_{12} in the ileum. The serum levels of iron, vitamin B_{12} and folic acid can all now be estimated and may indicate deficiency.

(i) Iron. If impaired absorption of iron is suspected then the serum levels can be repeated after oral treatment.
(ii) Vitamin B_{12}. The Schilling test is an index of vitamin B_{12} absorption. Radio-active labelled vitamin B_{12} is given by mouth and followed by measurement of the urinary and/or faecal radioactivity. In the diagnosis of pernicious anaemia the test can be repeated after giving the labelled vitamin together with the intrinsic factor.
(iii) Folic acid. Absorption is assessed either by serum levels after oral treatment or by comparison of the 24 hour urinary excretion of folic acid following successive oral and subcutaneous 5 mgm. doses. An excretion of less than 7.5 mgm. after the oral dose together with an excretion index of less than 75% indicates defective absorption.

The FIGLU test is a test of deficiency and not of absorption. In the absence of adequate folic acid oral histidine cannot be fully metabolised and the intermediate breakdown product (formiminoglutamic acid—FIGLU) is excreted in the urine and then measured.

9 LIVER BIOPSY (PERCUTANEOUS)

Samples of liver tissue can be obtained by means of percutaneous needle biopsy via the intercostal or subcostal routes after necessary preparation of in-patients. The Menghini and Vim-Silverman needles are those most commonly used in this country, the former being the simpler. The biopsy can be performed 'blind' or under direct vision during simultaneous peritoneoscopy.

Precautions:
1. Prior assessment of bleeding tendency (prothrombin time).
2. Blood grouping and availability of cross matched blood.
3. Aspiration of ascites if present.

Indications:
1. Diagnosis of diffuse lesions of the liver, i.e. infiltrations, chronic hepatitis and cirrhosis.
2. Diagnosis of nature of nodules in the liver, where secondary deposits are suspected, in order to prevent unnecessary laparotomy.

Suspected hydatid cysts should not be biopsied due to the risk of allergic reactions.

CHAPTER 20

DIET

The idea that diet is the essential therapeutic measure in the management of all varieties of gastro-intestinal upset is firmly entrenched in the lay mind, and is probably due to the frequent and undeniable association of many abdominal symptoms with eating. Up to a point this is a valid concept, since relief can be achieved in many cases by a temporary modification to the diet.

There are, however, two popular misconceptions:

1 That indifferent cooking is, in itself, the cause of digestive disease. In fact except for actual poisoning, unsuitable or ill-prepared food virtually never damages the 'digestion' (e.g. the evidence of concentration camps), although of course it may result in transient upsets.
2 That some people may be born with 'weak' digestions. The actual incidence of digestive enzyme deficiencies of congenital origin is very low and in any case many of them (e.g. achlorhydria) are entirely asymptomatic. The vast majority of patients who claim the misfortune of having been endowed with a 'weak' digestion are examples of purely functional disturbances and most have a psychogenic basis.

While in many cases of dyspepsia some modification or reorganisation of the diet is clearly a help, it is important to convince the patient that the aim should be to treat the primary cause so that the digestive tract can cope with a perfectly normal diet. In general therefore, diets should be permissive rather than restrictive.

The basic principles governing dietetic advice in the common gastro-intestinal disorders are outlined below:

PEPTIC ULCER

The essentials of dietary management are small, frequent, regular meals with something to eat every two to three hours ('between meal supplements'). Emphasis too should be laid on having a snack of milk and biscuits last thing at night.

The actual food content should be as near normal as possible but during exacerbations patients should be advised to avoid fried fats, strong spices, pickles, fizzy and very hot or cold fluids.

People on night shift work are particularly liable to symptoms and may need repeated advice. Medicinal antacids will be required to supplement the buffering action of food and this is further discussed in Chapter 4.

GALLBLADDER DISEASE

The stimulatory influence of dietary fat on the gallbladder is the basis of the fat-free diet that is so unnecessarily widely prescribed for biliary tract disorders.

It is of course important to reduce gallbladder activity to a minimum in acute cholecystitis and in the presence of gallstones because vesical contraction may possibly be dangerous as well as painful. On the other hand, in chronic or quiescent cholecystitis, stasis merely favours perpetuation of the disorder by encouraging further inspissation of bile.

There would be fewer disappointing results from cholecystectomy if only more attention were paid to the rationale of the conservative management of chronic cholecystitis, many instances of which would in any case be better considered as examples of simple biliary dyskinesia.

After warning the patient to expect a temporary excerbation of discomfort, a deliberate policy of drainage should be undertaken. Food should be palatable and as in peptic ulcer cases, taken in small quantities at frequent intervals. A gradually increasing quantity of fat should be included in each meal. Pure cream is often the most convenient and acceptable form since it is non-nauseating and can be taken in accurately measured increments as if it were medicine. Butter is perfectly permissible but cooked fats are best deferred until much later in the treatment.

Continuity of, and perseverance with, the régime is important since it may be some considerable time before full relief is achieved but eventual results can be very satisfactory. The co-incidental administration of cholagogues with a view to increasing the volume flow and reducing the viscosity of the bile is equally logical.

JAUNDICE

In the obstructive types of jaundice associated with biliary tract disease, a fat-free diet is undoubtedly advantageous as fats may provoke further symptoms but there is no necessity for restriction in the case of haemolytic jaundice. In the early stages of hepatocellular disorders, fats are not usually acceptable on account of nausea but can be safely introduced later.

REGIONAL ENTEROCOLITIS

During exacerbations of Crohn's disease the problem is essentially one of incipient, if not actual, bowel obstruction. In consequence a purely fluid diet is indicated. In view of the notorious chronicity of the condition this may have to be continued for some considerable time.

Even in the interim quiescent phases the lumen of sections of the intestine may be subject to a varying degree of constriction and therefore all indigestible, and especially non-absorbable, roughage should be excluded. Apart from this a full diet of normal constitution is both permissible and desirable. In actual fact, a low residue diet is far more applicable in Crohn's disease than it is in ulcerative colitis.

Some authorities have postulated the influence of a milk allergy in this condition and a trial of a milk-free diet may be considered.

DIVERTICULAR DISEASE

This acquired anatomical state is very commonly found by chance in elderly people without colonic symptoms and in these patients, no specific diet is indicated.

Apart from overt episodes of diverticulitis some patients experience more or less persistent discomfort in the left lower quadrant which is an expression of spasm in the pelvic or sigmoid colon. While the avoidance of irritant roughage in the diet is logical, it is important to ensure the presence of a reasonable quantity of soft residue material so as to maintain adequate bulk in the lower bowel. To this end sufficient green vegetables and salads should be included in the diet, always provided they are both tender and fresh. Tough greens or fibrous fruits are preferably avoided. Too refined a diet produces insufficient residue for smooth colonic activity and the resultant difficulty and irregularity with bowel actions invites provocation of the situation by means of purgatives.

Dietetic instructions should therefore not be too restrictive, although as mentioned above frank roughage is obviously best avoided.

IRRITABLE COLON SYNDROME (MUCOUS COLITIS: SPASTIC COLON)

This common disorder may or may not be a precursor of diverticular disease but the predominant feature from the symptomatic point of view is disordered muscular activity and spasm. Restoration of the normal integrated muscular activity should be the aim of treatment and in this the provision of bulk residue plays a major part.

There is no indication for a selective or restrictive diet in uncomplicated examples of this condition. It is far better dealt with by firm encouragement and persuasion to accept and persevere with a completely normal dietary intake.

ULCERATIVE COLITIS

In all phases of this destressingly protracted and profoundly debilitating condition, the outstanding dietetic requirement is that of a high calorie, high quality intake to compensate for the incessant drain of vital substances via the stool. The previously prevailing obsession with the necessity for a low residue diet was almost certainly in itself an added factor in the aggravation of the physical and psychological degradation of those suffering from the disease as the diet failed to match, let alone restore, the protein and mineral depletion. Even in the acute stage there is little, if any, convincing evidence that ordinary residue foods give rise to any aggravation of the local inflammation.

In the quiescent phases the diet can, and should, be perfectly normal, omitting only those particular constituents that the individual patient has found by experience provoke his symptoms. Mineral and vitamin supplements are advantageous, especially iron and the B complex.

As in Crohn's disease, although milk sensitivity is not the primary aetiological factor, a minority of patients benefit considerably from the institution of a milk-free diet.

GLUTEN INDUCED ENTEROPATHY (COELIAC DISEASE)

This is a highly specific condition and requires equally highly specific dietary measures. The inherent fault is a sensitivity of the small intestinal mucosal cell to the presence in the diet of the protein fraction gliadin and the exclusion of this from the diet is the first essential in treatment.

Gliadin, to which these patients are sensitive, is found principally in wheat and to a lesser extent in rye, barley and oats. Adequate diets using other cereals, especially corn and rice, can be constructed.

In treating these patients it is important to remember that a number of commercial flavourings and sauces also contain wheat gliadin and expert dietetic advice is required. Failure to do this may result in some of the apparent failures of treatment. Replacement of deficiencies of minerals and vitamins due to the malabsorption is also necessary.

EXAMINATION QUESTIONS

These questions have been set in the Medicine papers of the final examinations for medical degrees of the Universities of Cambridge (C), London (L), Oxford (O), West Indies and Ibadan and the final examinations for L.R.C.P. Lond., M.R.C.S. Eng. (Conj.).

1958

Discuss the diagnosis of abdominal colic. (Conj.)
Discuss the relationship between disease of the alimentary canal and anaemia. (Conj.)
A woman of 45 complains of difficulty in swallowing. Discuss the investigations and management. (Conj.)

1959

What disorders occur at the lower end of the oesophagus and how may they be distinguished? (Conj.)
What is the natural history of peptic ulcer?
What benefit can be expected from treatment? (Conj.)
Discuss the differential diagnosis and prognosis of acute hepatitis. (Conj.)

1960

Discuss the natural history and treatment of ulcerative colitis. (Conj.)
Describe the clinical manifestations of the malabsorption syndrome. Give an account of the causes and treatment of the condition. (Conj.)
A man aged 45 has had bad jaundice for a month. Discuss the differential diagnosis and investigations you would make. (L)

What do you understand by the term colon spasm? Discuss the causation of symptoms and treatment. (L)

Give an account of the treatment of obesity. (L)

1961

What are the complications of gastric ulcer and the diagnostic findings? (Conj.)

Give five complications of gall stones and in each case the symptoms and signs. (Conj.)

In what circumstances would you advise a patient with a duodenal ulcer to undergo a partial gastrectomy? What undesirable consequences may follow this operation? (Conj.)

1962

Describe the clinical features associated with hiatus hernia and discuss the management of this condition. (Conj.)

A man of 40 is found to have a mass in the right iliac fossa. How would you arrive at a diagnosis? (Conj.)

A woman of 50 complains of difficulty in swallowing. Discuss the differential diagnosis. (Conj.)

Describe the causes, symptoms and sequelae of gastro-oesophageal reflux. (L)

Discuss the differentiation between abdominal pain of organic and functional origin. (L)

Describe the investigations and discuss the differential diagnosis of a patient whose main complaint is diarrhoea. (Ibadan)

Describe the possible clinical features of the malabsorption syndrome. Discuss the investigation of this disorder. (West Indies)

1963

Give the most common symptom and therapeutic agent used in the treatment of infestation by:
 (a) ascaris lumbricoides
 (b) oxyuris vermicularis
 (c) taenia solium
 (d) giardia lamblia
 (e) ankylostoma duodenale. (Conj.)

Discuss the relation of anaemia to the G.I. tract. (Conj.)

What are the causes of cirrhosis of the liver? Describe the

pathological changes found. (Conj.)

Describe the ways in which disease of the liver may present. (Conj.)

In what circumstances would you advise surgical treatment for a patient suffering from duodenal ulcer ? What adverse effects may occur after recovering from the operation ? (Conj.)

Describe the clinical features of:
- (a) Crohn's disease
- (b) Duodenal ulcer
- (c) Ulcerative colitis
- (d) Carcinoma of the rectum
- (e) Carcinoma of the stomach
- (f) Gastro-colic fistula
- (g) Spastic colon
- (h) Achalasia of the cardia
- (i) Globus hystericus. (O)

Give the typical X-ray appearances of:
- (a) Chronic ulcerative colitis
- (b) Crohn's disease
- (c) Idiopathic steatorrhoea
- (d) Achalasia of the cardia. (O)

Discuss the causes of dysphagia in a female of 25. (C)

Discuss the management of a patient suffering from acute alcoholism. (C)

1964

Discuss the diagnosis and investigation of a patient with jaundice and fever. (Conj.)

What are the signs and symptoms of amoebiasis ? (Conj.)

Discuss the relationship of anaemia to disorders of the alimentary tract. (L)

Describe the symptoms, diagnosis and treatment of pyloric stenosis. (L)

Discuss the aetiology and treatment of hepatic failure. (L)

What are the causes of acute hepatitis? Discuss the value of tests of liver function. (L)

A middle-aged man is brought into hospital having vomited a large quantity of blood. Discuss the diagnosis and describe the immediate treatment of the patient. (L)

Write a short account of the clinical features and complications of cirrhosis of the liver. (Ibadan)

Describe the clinical features of the possible complications of peptic ulcer. Discuss briefly this management of these complications. (West Indies)

Discuss the pathophysiology of jaundice in a 56-year-old man. (West Indies)

What types of anaemia may occur in association with diseases of the G.I. tract? What is the mechanism of the anaemia in each type you describe? (C)

What advances of modern medicine have occurred since the end of the war in any one of these specialities:
(a) Gastro-enterology
(b) Neurology
(c) Renal disease.

1965

Discuss the treatment of portal cirrhosis and of its complications. (Conj.)

Define the treatment of the malabsorption syndrome and discuss the clinical manifestations. (Conj.)

Write an essay on overeating. (Conj.)

Write an essay on the malabsorption syndrome. (O)

Name three differences between infectious virus hepatitis and serum hepatitis and what measures can be used to prevent the spread of infectious virus hepatitis and serum hepatitis. What is the mortality rate and risk of permanent liver damage with each? What is the value in treatment of (a) rest; (b) diet and (c) cortico-steroids? (O)

Describe six tests used to diagnose the malabsorption syndrome. Explain how each is interpreted. (O)

List the main causes of impaired absorption of the small intestine (malabsorption syndrome). (C)

What are the hazards of gross obesity? (C)

How may carcinoma of the stomach present? (C)

Discuss the complications which may arise following surgical treatment for peptic ulcer, excluding those in the immediate post-operative period. (C)

A woman of 45 complains of intermittent pain in the right

iliac fossa for four months. What conditions must be considered in the differential diagnosis? (C)

A young man resident in this country has been suffering from diarrhoea for six months. Discuss the possible causes of the condition and any investigation of this patient. (C)

Discuss briefly the significance of:
  (a) Heartburn
  (b) Alternating constipation and diarrhoea
  (c) Pruritus ani (L)

Discuss the aetiology of peptic ulcer. (L)

What are the most important causes of the malabsorption syndrome? (L)

In what ways does cancer of the stomach present? Discuss the diagnosis. (L)

Describe the course of ulcerative colitis and its management. (L)

In what diseases may ulceration of the small bowel occur? (L)

Discuss the manifestations, investigations and management of pyloric stenosis in an elderly man (L)

What are the causes and complications of cirrhosis of the liver? (L)

Describe the aetiology, clinical picture and complications of pyloric obstruction. (L)

Describe the aetiology of peptic ulcer. (L)

Define the term malabsorption Syndrome and discuss the clinical manifestations. (Conj.)

Discuss the treatment of portal cirrhosis and of its complications. (Conj.)

1966
Discuss the diagnosis of jaundice in a man aged 60. (Conj.)

1967
Describe the treatment of Sonne dysentery and the management of an outbreak in hospital. (Conj.)

1968
Discuss the relationship of anaemia to disorders of the alimentary system. (Conj.)

RECOMMENDED BOOKS OF REFERENCE

BADENOCH J. & BROOKE B.N. eds (1965) *Recent Advances in Gastroenterology.* J. & A. Churchill, London.

BOCKUS H.L. *et al.* (1963, 1964, 1965) *Gastroenterology*, 2nd ed., in three volumes. W.B. Saunders, Philadelphia.

JONES, F. AVERY, GUMMER, J.W.P. & LENNARD-JONES, J.E. (1968) *Clinical Gastroenterology,* 2nd ed. Blackwell Scientific Publications, Oxford.

MCCONNELL R.B. (1966) *The Genetics of Gastro-intestinal Disorders.* Oxford University Press, London.

NAISH J.M. & READ A.E.A. (1965) *Basic Gastroenterology.* John Wright, Bristol.

SHERLOCK S. (1968) *Diseases of the Liver and Biliary System*, 4th ed. Blackwell Scientific Publications, Oxford.

TRUELOVE S.C. & REYNELL P.C. (1963) *Diseases of the Digestive System.* Blackwell Scientific Publications, Oxford.

INDEX

Abscess of liver
  amoebic 48
  bacterial 47,69
Absorption tests
  carbohydrate 190
  fat 189
  protein 190
  small intestinal 189
Accessory pancreatic rests 73
Achalasia of cardia 6
Achlorhydria
  chronic atrophic gastritis 16
  diarrhoea 132
  intestinal infection 84
Achylia gastrica 84,132
A.C.T.H. in ulcerative colitis 165
Adenoma, pancreas 79,80
Adenomatous polyps
  in Peutz-Jeghers syndrome 171
Adrenal, corticosteroids 42,78,146, 165,176
Afferent loop syndrome 33
Albumen, serum, and ascites 54,55
Alcohol
  cirrhosis 53
  liver toxin 52
  pancreatitis 76
  primary liver cancer 58
Allergic reactions
  causing diarrhoea 134
  Crohn's disease 142
Amanita phalloides 52
Amoebic dysentery 114
Amoebiasis, hepatic 48
Ampulla of Vater
  carcinoma of 71, 133
Amylase, serum 188
  in pancreatitis 77
Amyloidosis
  intestine 97

  liver 60
Anaemia, alimentary tract, causes of 101
Anaemia, iron deficiency
  in hiatus hernia 17
  post-gastrectomy 33
Anaemia, macrocytic
  in malabsorption syndrome 98
  post-gastrectomy 33
Angina, abdominal 93
Angiography 184
  carcinoma of pancreas 81
  ischaemic colitis 174
  mesenteric vascular occlusion 93
Ankylosing spondylitis
  in ulcerative colitis 162
Ankylostoma duodenale 123
Ankylostomiasis 123
Annular pancreas 73
Anorexia
  carcinoma of stomach 18
Antacids, use in peptic ulcer 30
Antibiotic, diarrhoea caused by 132
Antibiotics, use of
  in cholangitis 70
  in cholecystitis 60
  in cholera 112
  in Crohn's disease 146
  in food poisoning 108
  in hepatic coma 56
  in portal pyaemia 48
  in staphylococcal enterocolitis 109
  in syphilis 47
  in typhoid 110
  in ulcerative colitis 165
  in Weil's disease 46
  in Whipple's disease 176
Anticholinergic drugs 30,153

Index

Anticoagulants
  blood loss 102
  diarrhoea 132
Antimony
  in Bilharziasis 128
  liver toxin 52
Anxiety
  diarrhoea 137
  irritable colon 152
Aortography 184
  in ischaemic colitis 174
Appendicitis 149
Argentaffin cells 156,170
Argentaffinoma 170
Arsenic 52,132
Arthritis
  in ulcerative colitis 162
  in Whipple's disease 175
Ascariasis 125
Ascaris lumbricoides 123
Ascites, 54
Aspirin, and bleeding 35
Atresia, bile ducts 64
Atrophy, acute yellow 40
Augmented histamine test 186

Bacillary dysentery 113
Bacterial irritants, of bowel 131
Barium contrast studies 182
  enema 182
  follow-through 182
  swallow and meal 182
Barrett's ulcer 4
Beef tapeworm 120
Bile duct, atresia of 64
Bilharziasis
  hepatic 49
    carcinoma 58
    cirrhosis 53,128
  intestinal 127
Biliary
  calculi 64
  cirrhosis 56
    in cholangitis 69
  tract 64-71
    carcinoma 58
    cholelithiasis 64
    congenital anomalies 64
    infections 66

    tumours 70
Bilious vomiting 33
Bilirubin
  excretion, tests of 186
  calculi 64
Biopsy
  gastric 185
    in carcinoma of the stomach 18
  liver 191
    in Bilharziasis 50
    in cirrhosis 55
    in glandular fever 43
    in infective hepatitis 42
    in primary cancer 58
    in secondary deposits 59
  small intestine 185
    in carcinoma 92
    in disaccharidase deficiency 91
    in giardiasis 116
    in gluten induced enteropathy 89
    in malabsorption syndrome 99
    in tropical sprue 90
    in Whipple's disease 176
  rectal 185
    in carcinoma 155
    in Hirschsprung's disease 154
    in regional enterocolitis 145
    in ulcerative colitis 163
    in Whipple's disease 176
Bleeding
  frank rectal 36
  gastrointestinal
    acute 34
    chronic 102
Blood transfusion 37
Botulism 108
British anti-lewisite 52
Bromsulphthalein excretion test 188
Butazolidin, and bleeding 35

Caeruloplasmin 61
Calculi, biliary 64
Candida albicans 117
Carbenoxolone sodium 31
Carbohydrate metabolism, tests of 187
Carbon tetrachloride 52
Carcinoid tumours 156,170

Index

Carcinoma
  ampulla of Vater 71,133
  colon 154
  gallbladder 70
  liver 58
  oesophagus 7
  pancreas 80
  peptic ulcer, association with 29
  rectum 154
  small intestine 92
  stomach 17,29
Casoni test 51,123
Central venous pressure, measurement of 37
Cestodes 120–123
Chaga's disease 6
Chelating agents
  in haemochromatosis 62
  in Wilson's disease 62
Chemical bowel irritants 132
Chloroform 52
Chloroquin 49
Chlorpromazine 52
Chlorpropamide 52
Cholagogues 69,194
Cholangiography, intravenous 183
  gall stones 66
Cholangioma 58
Cholangitis, ascending 47
Cholecystectomy 68
Cholecystitis
  acute 66
  chronic 67
Cholecystography, oral 183
  in cholecystitis 68
Cholelithiasis 64
Cholera 112
Cholestatic jaundice 51
Cholesterol, gallstones 64
Chromaffin cells 170
Cirrhosis 9,53
  alcohol and 53
  biliary 56
  in cholangitis 69
  in haemochromatosis 53
  Laennec's 9,53
  multilobular 9,53
  portal 9,53
  portal hypertension in 9,54
  post viral 56
  primary cancer in 58
  in ulcerative colitis 162
  varices, oesophageal, in 9
  in Wilson's disease 53
Clostridium Botulinum 108
Coeliac disease 87,96
  diet in 196
Colchicine 132
Colectomy, in ulcerative colitis 166
Colitis
  distal 158
  extensive 158
  ischaemic 173
  left-sided 158
  mucous 152
  nervous 152
  proximal 158
  total 158
  ulcerative 158–166
Colloidal gold reaction 187
Colon 148–158
  carcinoma 154
  disorders, classification of 148
  diverticula 150
  dyskinesia 152
  infections 148
  irritable, syndrome of 152
  spastic 152
  tumours 154
Coma, hepatic 56
Congenital anomalies
  gallbladder 64
  oesophagus 10
  pancreas 72
Constipation
  in carcinoma of colon 155
  in Hirschsprung's disease 154
  in lead poisoning 132
  in ulcerative colitis 161,164
Copper metabolism 161
Corrosive oesophagitis 1
Crohn's disease 87,142–147
  aetiology 142
  clinical features 143
  diarrhoea in 134
  diet in, 194
  investigations 144
  pathology 142
  treatment 145
Curling's ulcer 26

Index

Cushing's ulcer 26
Cystic fibrosis, pancreas 73
Cysts
  air, of intestine 174
  hydatid, of liver 50,122
Cytology, exfoliative gastric 19

Deep X-ray, as bowel irritant 132
Dehydrogenase, lactic 188
Desferrioxamine 62
Diabetes mellitus
  diarrhoea in 136
  in pacreatitis 79
Diaphragm, eventration of 5
Diarrhoea 130–141
  causes of 130
  definition 130
  differential diagnosis 139
  lienteric 132
  post-vagotomy 33
  spurious 138
  treatment 140
Dibothriocephalus latus 121
Diet 192–196
  in diverticular disease 152,194
  in irritable colon syndrome 195
  in gallbladder disease 69,193
  in jaundice 194
  in peptic ulcer 29,193
  in regional enterocolitis 145, 194
  in ulcerative colitis 195
Dietary fat, absorption of 189
Digestive secretion defects
  diarrhoea 132
Digitalis 132
Disaccharidase deficiencies 90
  estimation 91
Disaccharides, absorption of 190
Diverticula
  colonic 150
  duodenal 85
  gastric 20
  Meckel's 86
  oesophageal 11
  small intestinal 85
Drugs
  as bowel irritants 132
  as causes of bleeding 35
  as liver toxins 51

Dumping syndrome 33
Duodenal
  diverticula 85
  ulcer 26
Dye excretion tests 188
Dysentery
  amoebic 114
  bacillary 113
Dyskinesia
  biliary 193
  of colon 152
Dyspepsia 22
  nervous 25
Dysphagia
  in carcinoma 8
  in oesophagitis 2
  sideropaenic 3

Echinococcus, taenia 50,122
Ectopic gastric mucosa 167
Electroencephalography
  in liver disease 55,56
Emetine, use of
  in amoebic dysentery 115
  in amoebic hepatitis 49
Endoscopy 179
Enterobiasis 124
Enterobius vermicularis 123
Enterocolitis
  phlegmonous 109
  pseudomembranous 109
  regional (Crohn's disease) 87, 142–147
  staphylococcal 109
Enzymes, intramucosal, deficiencies
  of 90
  serum 77,81
    as tests of liver function 188
Erosions, stomach 14
Erythema nodosum
  in ulcerative colitis 162
Eventration, of diaphragm 5
Examination questions 197

Faecal fat, estimation of 189
  in malabsorption syndrome 98
Faeces, examination of 179
  occult blood test 179

Index

Familial polyposis 156,172
Fat absorption, tests of 189
Fibrocystic disease of pancreas 73
FIGLU test 191
Fish tapeworm 121
Fissure, in ulcerative colitis 161
Fistula
  in regional enterocolitis 144
  in ulcerative colitis 161
Flatulence 22,23
Flocculation tests 187
Folic acid
  absorption, tests of 191
  in atrophic gastritis 17
  impaired assimilation, cases of 103
  in malabsorption syndrome 98
  treatment with 105
Food poisoning 107
Foreign bodies, in oesophagus 12
Formiminoglutamic acid 191
Function tests 186
  gastric 186
  hepatic 186
  pancreatic 188
  small intestinal 189
Fungus, infections, of intestine 117

Gall bladder 64–71
  agenesis 64
  anomalies 64
  bilobed 64
  carcinoma 70
  diverticula 64
  malposition 64
Gallstones 64–66,67
  carcinoma of gallbladder 70
  cholecystitis 66,67
Gastrectomy, partial
  carcinoma 17
  peptic ulcer 32
Gastric
  biopsy 185
  cooling 38
  function tests 186
    in carcinoma 19
    in peptic ulcer 29
    in Zollinger-Ellison syndrome 169
  lavage 10
  mucosa, ectopic 167
Gastrin, in Zollinger-Ellison syndrome 169
Gastritis 14
  acute erosive 14
  carcinoma in 17
  chronic atrophic 16
  chronic hypertrophic 16
  subacute inflammatory 15
Gastroduodenitis 15
Gastroenteritis 106
  in infancy 118
Gastroenterostomy, for peptic ulcer 32
Gastrointestinal bleeding
  acute 34–38
  chronic 101–105
Gastroscopy 180
  carcinoma stomach 18
  gastritis 16
  peptic ulcer 29
  Peutz-Jeghers syndrome 172
Giardiasis 115
Glandular fever, liver involvement 43
Gliadin 87
Globus hystericus 3
Gluten induced enteropathy 87
  diet in 196
Gold, liver toxin 52
Granular proctitis 158
  diarrhoea in 139

Haematemesis
  oseophageal varices 9
  peptic ulcer 28,34
Haematemesis, and melaena 34–38
  common causes 34
  clinical features 34
  diagnosis of source 35
  investigations 35
  treatment 37
Haemochromatosis 61
  carcinoma of liver 53
  cirrhosis 53
Haemopoietic factors
  impaired assimilation of 102

Index

Haemorrhage, gastrointestinal
  acute 34–38
  chronic 101–105
Haemorrhagic pancreatitis 75
Haemorrhoids 157
Heller's operation 7
Helminth infestations 120–129
  classification 120
Hepatic biopsy, percutaneous 191
Hepatic coma 10,55
Hepatic function tests 42,43,54,57, 186–188
Hepatitis
  infective 40
  post-viral 56
  serum 43
  toxic 52
  viral 40,43
Hepato-allergens 51
Hepatolenticular degeneration 61
  cirrhosis 53
Hepatoma 58
Hepatotoxins 51
Hereditary telangiectasia
  as a cause of blood loss 101
Hernia, hiatus 4
Heterotopic pancreas 73,168
Hiatus hernia 4
  classification 4
Hirschsprung's disease 153
Histalog test 186
Histamine, augmented, test 186
Hodgkin's disease, liver 59
Hookworm 123
Hourglass deformity, stomach 28
Hydatid cysts 50,122
Hydroxycobalamin
  absorption tests 191
  atrophic gastritis 17
  diverticulosis 86
  impaired assimilation 103
  malabsorption syndrome 98
  treatment with 105
Hyperparathyroidism
  pancreatitis 76
Hypertension, portal venous 9,54
Hyperthyroidism
  as a cause of diarrhoea 136
Hypertrophic pyloric stenosis 19

Indigestion 22–25
  differential diagnosis 24
  investigations 25
  types 22
Idiopathic steatorrhoea 87,96
  diet in 196
Ileorectal anastomosis in ulcerative colitis 166
Ileus, paralytic 94
Infarction, bowel 93,173
Infections
  as cause of diarrhoea 131
  liver
    bacterial 47,48
    spirochaetal 45
    viral 40
  intestinal 106–119
    bacterial 106
    classification 106
    fungal 117
    protozoal 114
    viral 116
Infectious mononucleosis, of liver 43
Infestations
  Helminth, intestinal 120
  liver 48
Infiltrations, of liver 59
Insulinoma 79,80
Insulin secreting tumours of pancreas 79,80
Intestinal
  bleeding
    acute 34–38
    chronic 101–105
  infarction 93,173
  infections 106–119
  infestations 120–129
  malabsorption 96–100
  obstruction 94
Intussusception, of small intestine 94
Investigation techniques 178–191
Iridocyclitis, in ulcerative colitis 162
Iron
  absorption 191
  impaired assimilation, causes of 103
  treatment with 105

Index

Iron-deficiency anaemia
  chronic atrophic oesophagitis 3
  hiatus hernia 17
  malabsorption syndrome 98
  oesophageal web 3
  post-gastrectomy 33
Irritable colon, syndrome 152
  diet in 195
Irritants, as cause of diarrhoea 131
Ischaemic colitis 93,173
Islet-cell tumours, of pancreas 79
  diarrhoea 137
Isonicotinic acid hydrazine 52
Isotopes, radioactive, use of 184
  blood loss 184
  fat absorption 189
  liver tumours 58
  pancreatic carcinoma 81

Jaundice
  biliary cirrhosis 57
  carcinoma of ampulla of Vater 71
  cholangitis 70
  cholecystitis 68
  cholestatic 51
  chronic pancreatitis 79
  cirrhosis 54
  drugs, causing 52
  gall stones 65
  glandular fever 43
  infective hepatitis 42
  leptospirosis 45
  steroid treatment of 42
  syphilis 46
  yellow fever 44
Jejunal diverticulosis 85
  malabsorption syndrome 96
Juvenile polyps 156

Kayser-Fleischer ring 61
Kwashiorkor
  cirrhosis 53
Lactase deficiency 90
  diarrhoea 135
  investigation of 190
Lactic dehydrogenase 188
Laennec's cirrhosis 53
Lead poisoning 132

Leptospirosis of liver 45
Leukaemia, liver involvement 60
Lienteric diarrhoea 132
Lipase intestinal, inactivation of 169
  pancreatitis 77
  serum 188
Lipoidoses, of liver 60
Liver 39–63
  abscess
    amoebic 48
    bacterial 47,69
  amoebiasis 48
  amyloidosis 60
  Bilharziasis 49
  biopsy 191
    in Bilharziasis 50
    in cirrhosis 55
    in glandular fever 43
    in infective hepatitis 42
    in primary cancer 58
    in secondary deposits 59
  cirrhosis 9,53
    alcohol and 53
    biliary 56
    in cholangitis 69
    in haemochromatosis 53
    Laennec's 9,53
    multilobular 9,53
    portal 9,53
    portal hypertension 9,54
    post viral 56
    primary cancer in 58
    in ulcerative colitis 162
    varices oesophageal, in 9
    in Wilson's disease 53
  cysts, hydatid 50, 122
  disorders, classification of 39
  "flap" 54
  function tests 186–188
    in biliary cirrhosis 57
    in portal cirrhosis 54
    in glandular fever 43
    in infective hepatitis 42
  glandular fever 43
  haemochromatosis 61
  infections 40
    bacterial 47
    spirochaetal 45
    viral 40
  infestations 48

infiltrations   59
leptospirosis   45
leukaemia   60
lipoidoses   60
"palms"   54
poisons   51
porphyria   62
reticuloses   59
sarcoidosis   60
syphilis   46
systemic lupus erythematosus   60
tuberculosis   48
tumours, primary
  benign   58
  malignant   58
tumours, secondary   59
Weil's disease   45
yellow fever   44
Lupus erythematosus, of liver   60
Lymphangiectasia, congenital   97
Lymphatic obstruction
  in Whipple's disease   175
Lymphoma
  of small intestine   92
Malabsorption syndrome   96–100
  causes of   96
  clinical features of   97
  diarrhoea in   134
  differential diagnosis of   99
  gluten induced enteropathy   88
  investigations in   98
  small intestinal diverticulosis   86
  treatment of   100
  tropical sprue   90
Mallory-Weiss syndrome   12
Maltase deficiency   90
  investigation of   190
Meckel's diverticulum   86
  ectopic gastric mucosa in   168
  peptic ulcer in   26
Meconium ileus
  cystic fibrosis   74
Megacolon
  Hirschsprung's disease   153
  toxic, in ulcerative colitis   162
Megaoesophagus   6
Melaena
  oesophageal varices   9
  peptic ulcer   28

Melaena, and haematemesis   34–38
  common causes of   34
  clinical features   34
  diagnosis of source   35
  investigations   35
  treatment   37
Menetrier's disease   16
Mercury   52,132
Mesenteric adenitis   50
  vascular occlusion   93,173
    diarrhoea in   135
Microvilli, abnormalities of in gluten
    induced enteropathy   88
Midgut ischaemia   93
Milk antibodies   135
  protein diarrhoea   135
Moniliasis   117
Monosaccharides, absorption of   190
Motility studies   185
Mucous colitis   152
  diet in   195
Mucoviscidosis   73
Multiple familial polyposis   156

Nausea   23
Necator Americanus   123
Necrosing pancreatitis   75
Nematodes   123–127
Neomycin   56,132
Nervous colitis   152
  dyspepsia   25

Obstruction, small intestine   94
Occult blood in faeces   104,109
Oesophageal varices   9,34,54
Oesophagitis acute (corrosive)   1
  chronic atrophic   3
  classification of   1
  recurrent reflux   3
  subacute   2
Oesophageal balloon   10
Oesophagoscopy   179
  carcinoma   8
  foreign bodies   13
  varices   10
Oesophagus   1–13
  carcinoma   7
  congenital anomalies   10

Index

diverticula 11
ectopic gastric mucosa in 168
foreign bodies 12
peptic ulcer 4
perforation 12
stricture 2,10
trauma 11
"web" 3
Osteomalacia
  malabsorption syndrome 99
  postgastrectomy 33
Osteoporosis
  malabsorption syndrome 99
  post-gastrectomy 33
Oxyuris vermicularis 123

Palms, liver 54
Pancreas 72–82
  annular 73
  congenital anomalies 72
  cystic fibrosis of 74
  disorders, classification of 72
  duct obstruction 76,133
  duct variations 72
  fistula 73
  heterotopic 73,168
  inflammation 75
  inherited disease 73
  lithiasis 78
  pseudocyst 75
  rests, accessory 73
  trauma 75
  tumours 79
Pancreatectomy
  carcinoma 82
  pancreatitis 79
Pancreatic enzymes, treatment with 79
Pancreatic insufficiency
  as cause of diarrhoea 133
Pancreatitis
  acute 75
  chronic 78
    diarrhoea in 133
  haemorrhagic 75
  necrotising 75
  subacute relapsing 78
Pancreozymin 79,179
Papilloma, villous 156

Paralytic ileus 94
Paratyphoid 111
Paterson-Kelly syndrome 3
Penicillamine 61
Pentagastrin 186
Peptic ulcer 26–33
  acute 26
  aetiology 27
  carcinoma in 29
  chronic (persistent) 27
  classification 26
  clinical features 27
  complications 28
  haemorrhage 28
  in hiatus hernia 26
  in jejunum 26
  in Meckel's diverticulum 26
  in oesophagus 4,26
  investigations 29
  penetrating 28
  perforation 28
  post-operative complications 32
  sites of occurrence 26
  stenosis 28
  subacute (recurrent) 26
  treatment, medical 29
    surgical 32
Percutaneous
  biopsy, liver 191
  cholangiography
    in biliary cirrhosis 57
Perforation, peptic ulcer 28
Pericholangitis
  in ulcerative colitis 162
Peritoneoscopy 180
Pernicious anaemia
  carcinoma stomach 17
  chronic atrophic gastritis 16
Peutz-Jeghers syndrome 171
Pharyngeal web 3
Phenindione 52
Phenylbutazone 52
Phlebotomy 62
Phosphatase, alkaline 188
"Piles" 157
Pigmentation
  in Peutz-Jeghers syndrome 171
Plain abdominal film, X-ray 181
Plummer-Vinson syndrome 3

Pneumatosis cystoides intestinalis 174
Poisons, liver 51
Polyposis, coli 172
  multiple familial 156,172
Polyps, adenomatous of colon 156
  adenomatous in Peutz-Jeghers syndrome 171
  juvenile 156
  pseudo- 159
Pork tapeworm 120
Porphyria 62
Portal hypertension 9,54
  pyaemia 47
  venography 184
Portal-systemic encephalopathy 56
Portal vein, obstruction 9
  thrombosis 9
Post-gastrectomy syndromes 32
  anaemia 102
Post-necrotic scarring 56
Pressure studies 186
Proctitis 158
Proctoscopy 181
Proctosigmoiditis 158
Protein
  absorption
    in hepatic coma 56
    tests of 190
  metabolism, hepatic
    tests of 187
Pruritus
  biliary cirrhosis 57
  cholangitis 70
  threadworms 124
Pyaemia, portal 47
Pyloric stenosis
  hypertrophic 19
  in peptic ulcer 29
Pyloroplasty 32
Pyoderma gangrenosum 162

Quinine, diarrhoea 132

Radiation, as bowel irritant 132
Radioactive isotopes, use of 184
  blood loss 184
  fat absorption 189

liver tumours 58
  pancreatic carcinoma 81
Radiography, use of 181
"Radio-pills" 186
Radiotherapy 8
Rectum
  biopsy
    in carcinoma 155
    in Hirschsprung's disease 154
    in regional enterocolitis 145
    in ulcerative colitis 163
  carcinoma 154
  disorders of 148–158
  frank bleeding from 36
  haemorrrhoids 156
  tumours 154
Reflux oesophagitis 3
Regional enteritis 142
Regional enterocolitis 87, 142–147
  aetiology 142
  clinical features 143
  diarrhoea in 134
  diet in 194
  investigations 144
  pathology 142
  treatment 145
Reticuloses, of liver 59
Rolling hernia 4
Rose Bengal 188
Roundworms 125

Sacroiliitis, in ulcerative colitis 162
Salicylazosulphapyridine (Salazopyrin) 165
Salmonella, food-poisoning 108
  paratyphosum A and B 111
  typhosum 110
Sarcoidosis, liver 60
Sarcoma, liver 58
  small intestine 92
  stomach 19
Scanning, radioisotopic 184
  liver 58
  pancreas 81
Schilling test 104,191
Schistosomiasis
  hepatic 49
    cirrhosis in 53
  intestinal 127

Scintillation counting 184
Scleroderma 176
Secretin 79,189
Sengstaken, oesophageal tube 10
Septicaemia
  cholangitis 69
Serotonin 170
Shellfish, causing diarrhoea 135
Shigella, shiga 113
  sonnei 113
Sideropaenic dysphagia 3,7
Sigmoidoscopy 181
  in amoebic dysentery 115
  in carcinoma rectum 155
  in diverticulitis 151
  in familial polyposis coli 172
  in Peutz-Jegher's syndrome 172
  in pneumatosis cystoides intestinalis 174
  in ulcerative colitis 163
Skip lesions (Crohn's) 143
Sliding hernia 4
Small intestine 83-95
  absorption tests 189
  biopsy 185
    in carcinoma 92
    in disaccharidase deficiency 91
    in giardiasis 116
    in gluten induced enteropathy 89
    in malabsorption syndrome 99
    in tropical sprue 90
    in Whipple's disease 176
  Crohn's disease 87
  disorders of, classification 83
  diverticula 85
  infections 84
  inflammatory disease 87
  mucosal enzyme disorders 87
  obstruction 94
  tumours 91
Spastic colon 152
  diet in 195
Spider naevi 54
Spurious diarrhoea 138
Staphylococcal enterocolitis 109
  food poisoning 108
Steatorrhoea
  in biliary cirrhosis 57
  in cystic fibrosis 74
  idiopathic 87
  in malabsorption syndrome 98
  in pancreatitis 79
  in systemic sclerosis 176
  tests for 189
  in Zollinger-Ellison syndrome 169
Steroid, hormones, and bleeding 35
  hormones, use of
    in hepatitis 42
    in pancreatitis 78
    in regional enterocolitis 146
    in ulcerative colitis 165
    in Whipple's disease 176
Stomach 14-21
  atrophy 16
  carcinoma 17
  cooling 38
  disorders of, common 14
  diverticula 20
  erosions 14
  hourglass deformity 28
  hypertrophy, of mucosa 16
  inflammation 14
  peptic ulcer 16-23
  sarcoma 19
  stenosis, hypertrophic pyloric 19
  tumours 19
  volvulus 20
Stool
  culture 179
    in cholera 112
    in food poisoning 108
    in staphylococcal enteritis 109
    in typhoid 110
  examination 179
  "rice-water", in cholera 112
Stricture, ischaemic of colon 173
  oesophageal 2,10,176
  in regional enteritis 144
  in ulcerative colitis 159
String sign 144
Strongyloides stercoralis 123,126
Strongyloidiasis 123,126
Sucrase deficiency 90
  investigation of 190
Syphilis of liver 46
  cirrhosis 53
Systemic sclerosis, progressive 176

Index

Taenia echinococcus 50,122
  saginata 120
  solium 120
Tapeworms 120
  beef 120
  fish 121
  pork 120
Telangiectasia, multiple hereditary as a cause of blood loss 101
Telemetering capsules 186
Terminal ileitis 87,142
Testosterone
  haemochromatosis 61
  liver toxin 52
Thrush 118
Thymol turbidity reaction 187
Thyrotoxicosis, diarrhoea in 136
Tolbutamide 52
Toxic hepatitis 52
Transaminase, serum 188
Transfusion, blood 37
Trematodes 127
Trichinella spiralis 123,127
Trichinosis 123,127
Trichuriasis 126
Trichuris trichiura 123
Tropical sprue 89
Tubeless test meal 186
Tuberculosis, of liver 48
Tumours
  carcinoid 156,170
  colon 154
  gallbladder 70
  islet cell 79
  liver 58
  oesophagus 10
  pancreas 79
  rectum 154
  small intestine 191
  stomach 17
Typhoid 110

Ulcer, Barrett's 4
  Cushing's 26
  Curling's 26
  peptic 26–33
Ulcerative colitis 158–166
  aetiology 159
  classification 158
  clinical features 159
  complications 161
  definition 158
  diarrhoea in 134
  diet in 164, 195
  investigations 163
  pathology 159
  psychological aspects 162
  treatment 163

Vagotomy
  in achalasia 7
  diarrhoea following 137
  peptic ulcer 32
Varices, oesophageal 9,34,54
Vascular, occlusion, mesenteric 93,173
Vater, ampulla of, carcinoma 71,133
Venesection, in haemochromatosis 62
Venography, portal 184
Villi, intestinal, abnormalities of
  in gluten induced enteropathy 88
  in malgnant disease 92
  in tropical sprue 89
  in Whipple's disease 175
Villous papilloma 156
Virus infections, intestine 116
  liver 40
Vitamin B_{12}
  absorption, tests of 191
  in atrophic gastritis 17
  impaired assimilation, causes of 103
  in malabsorption syndrome 98
  in small intestinal diverticulosis 86
  treatment with 105
Volvulus, small intestine 94
  stomach 20
Vomit, examination of 178

Weil's disease 45
Whipple's disease 175
Widal reaction 111

Wilson's disease 61
  cirrhosis 53

Xanthomata, in biliary cirrhosis 57
Xylose absorption test 190
  in malabsorption syndrome 98

Yellow fever 44
  vaccine 44

Zinc sulphate reaction 187
Zollinger-Ellison syndrome 80, 169
  peptic ulcer in 26